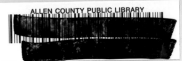
THE EYE LASER MIRACLE

THE COMPLETE GUIDE TO BETTER VISION

THE
EYE
LASER
MIRACLE

THE COMPLETE GUIDE
TO BETTER VISION

ANDREW I. CASTER, M.D.

BALLANTINE BOOKS
NEW YORK

A Ballantine Book
The Ballantine Publishing Group

Copyright © 1997, 2001 by Andrew I. Caster, M.D., F.A.C.S.

All rights reserved under International and Pan-American Copyright Conventions. Published in the United States by The Ballantine Publishing Group, a division of Random House, Inc., New York, and simultaneously in Canada by Random House of Canada Limited, Toronto. Originally published in different form by The Ballantine Publishing Group, a division of Random House, Inc., in 1997.

Ballantine and colophon are registered trademarks of Random House, Inc.

www.randomhouse.com/BB/

Library of Congress Card Number: 00-109196

ISBN 0-345-44383-7

Artwork: Cartoon drawings by Jay Jackson; scanning electron micrograph courtesy of IBM; laser light drawing by Stephen F. Gordon; all other artwork courtesy of Blausen Medical Communications.

Cover photo © Silverstock/Stock Connection

Manufactured in the United States of America

First Revised Trade Edition: January 2001

10 9 8 7 6 5 4 3 2 1

CONTENTS

AUTHOR'S NOTE

Throughout this book, statistics were frequently taken from the guidebooks for physicians published by laser manufacturers and are identified as follows:

(a) Summit Technology, "Apex Excimer Laser System Physician Information";

(b) VISX, "Professional Use Information Manual."

Other statistics have been taken from:

(c) CRS LASIK FDA Ophthalmic Panel Presentation.

INTRODUCTION

Seeing well without glasses and contact lenses is the dream of millions of Americans. Modern medical science has enabled this dream to come true.

Excimer laser surgery is the extremely popular treatment for nearsightedness, farsightedness, and astigmatism, and it can permanently eliminate the need to wear glasses or contact lenses for distance vision. The original version of excimer laser treatment, PRK (photorefractive keratectomy), uses a laser beam to reshape the surface of the cornea (the outer layer of the eye) to diminish nearsightedness, farsightedness, and astigmatism. Another kind of excimer laser treatment, LASIK (laser in-situ keratomileusis), reduces nearsightedness, farsightedness, and astigmatism by applying the laser treatment to the deep portion of the cornea. Both procedures are quick—usually taking no more than five to ten minutes—and painless. The results, as patients and their doctors will tell you, are impressive.

• Stacy, a forty-year-old music publisher, had been wearing corrective lenses since she was in the sixth grade. For thirty years, she couldn't get out of bed in the morning without putting on her glasses. "As a child, I would play a game: If I had three wishes, what would they be? 20/20 vision, 20/20 vision, 20/20 vision. It's always been the first thing I would change about my life." Three weeks after having LASIK, Stacy's vision had improved from 20/800 to 20/20. "Your confidence level goes up," she said. "It's not so much the way you look. It's the way you feel. I feel so good about myself."

• Ted was so nearsighted and astigmatic that he could barely see his hand in front of his face without glasses. Before having surgery, he went sailing with his nine-year-old son. The boom knocked Ted's glasses off. He grabbed them just before they landed in the water. Without them, he couldn't see the shore. That close call convinced him that it was time to get rid of his glasses. LASIK surgery gave him 20/25 vision. "What's dramatic," the forty-eight-year-old teacher said, "is being able to open your eyes in the morning and actually being able to see."

• Ethan, a thirty-two-year-old actor with 20/800 vision, had been wearing contact lenses for years. By the end of the day, his eyes were tired and red. Now that he's had PRK, he has 20/25 vision in the left eye and 20/20 in the right. "It's one less worry in my life," he said. "It's made my life a little less complicated. I don't have to put in contacts or get my glasses. I just feel freer."

• LASIK surgery gave Diane, a forty-five-year-old physician's assistant, a newfound sense of freedom, too. Before LASIK, she couldn't clearly see her feet when she was in the shower. Now she's taking rock-climbing lessons with her twelve-year-old daughter, something she would never do when she had to wear glasses or contacts. "I always believed I was entitled to see well," she said. With 20/30 vision in her left eye and 20/40 in the right, she finally does. "It's within a person's grasp. It's wonderful that technology has come this far."

However, excimer laser surgery is not for everyone, and it is not risk free. It is also not 100 percent effective for all patients.

Radial keratotomy, invented in 1973, was the first technique used to enable people to see without glasses or contact lenses. Now, over twenty-five years later, dramatically advanced techniques using lasers controlled by computers perform even more accurate treatments. Because of the ease of treatment and the accuracy of results, excimer laser procedures have become one of the most commonly performed surgeries in the United States. More than one million excimer laser procedures will be performed this year in the United States alone, and a similar number in the rest of the world.

I have written this book to explain to you the pros and cons of excimer laser surgery and to present other information necessary to help you make an informed decision. Part I provides basic information and should be read by everyone contemplating this procedure, Part II provides additional information for those who want to know more, and the Afterword describes my own experience as a patient having excimer laser vision correction.

Part I includes simple background information, the characteristics of a good candidate for excimer laser treatment, and how the procedure works. Part I also describes the procedure itself, from the presurgical consultation through the postoperative phase. Finally, it points out what results you can expect and what can go wrong.

The last section of Part I answers the most commonly asked questions about excimer laser eye surgery. All readers will find this particularly useful.

Part II is for people who require additional information, a behind-the-scenes exploration. It describes what a laser is, the role of the FDA in evaluating the laser procedure, alternatives to excimer laser treatment, as well as possible future developments.

This book provides the consumer with important background information concerning excimer laser treatment. Every effort has been made to provide accurate information and a balanced viewpoint, but the accuracy of information cannot be guaranteed. When statistics are given, they are usually taken from FDA supervised studies, but multiple studies conducted in different fashions produce varying statistics. The decision to have excimer laser treatment must be based upon an evaluation and critical discussion with your doctor of your specific medical condition, lifestyle, and desires.

PART
I

||||||||||||||||||||||||||||

BASIC
INFORMATION

—

EVERYONE
SHOULD READ
THIS

|||||||||||||||||||||||||||

THE
SURGERY IS EASY

Excimer laser treatment is a very easy procedure to undergo. No injections are needed, and there is no pain during the procedure. These are the steps you will experience:

1. Your doctor will measure your eyes to determine your amount of nearsightedness, farsightedness, and astigmatism. During this presurgical consultation, your doctor will complete a thorough examination of the health of your eyes and discuss the procedure in detail with you.

2. The excimer laser will be calibrated and tested for accuracy.

3. The correction desired for your eye will be entered into the laser's computer.

4. The computer will determine the specific set of excimer laser pulses to apply.

5. You will be brought into the laser room and asked to lie down.

6. A patch will be placed over the eye not having the procedure.

7. Anesthetic eyedrops will be placed in your eye. No injections or IVs are needed.

8. Your eyelid will be held open with a small speculum, which causes no pain.

9. You will be asked to look at a small blinking light.

10. In LASIK, the flap will be created with the keratome. In PRK, the doctor will wipe away the most superficial layer of the cornea.

11. You will hear a clicking noise, the sound of the laser.

12. The blinking light will get hazy as the treatment progresses.

13. The treatment will usually take less than sixty seconds of laser time.

14. Eyedrops will be placed in your eye. In some cases, a temporary contact lens will be placed in your eye as well.

15. You will sit up and rest for a few minutes before going home. Your stay in the treatment room has lasted about five to ten minutes.

Sounds easy, doesn't it? And it is. But how accurate are the results? What can go wrong? Are you a suitable candidate for excimer laser surgery, or should you consider alternatives? These questions will be addressed shortly. First, we will examine the biology and mechanics of the eye.

||||||||||||||||||||||||||||

HOW DOES
THE EYE WORK?

Just like a camera, the eye works by focusing light rays. Light entering the eye first passes through a transparent layer called the cornea. The cornea acts as a lens by focusing the light. Located behind the cornea is another lens, known as the crystalline lens, that further focuses the light to make a clear image on the retina at the back of the eye. Finally, the image is transmitted to the brain by the optic nerve.

Just as a camera cannot produce a clear photograph if the incoming light is not focused precisely onto the film, so the eye cannot produce clear vision if the cornea and crystalline lens do not focus the light precisely onto the retina.

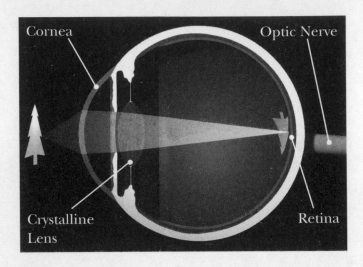

The eye is very similar to a camera. Light rays are focused by the cornea and crystalline lens. The focus must be accurate in order to obtain a clear image.

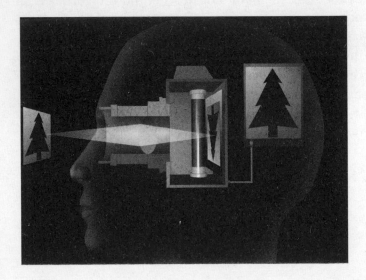

||||||||||||||||||||||||||||

COMMON
VISION PROBLEMS

The most common vision problem is the inability to focus incoming light precisely onto the retina. The result is blurred vision.

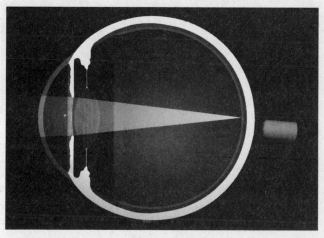

Normal eye

There are four types of focusing errors:

Nearsightedness. Nearsighted people see near objects better than those farther away. In nearsightedness (also known as myopia), light rays from distant objects are focused not onto the retina but in front of the retina. Nearsightedness occurs because the cornea and the crystalline lens together have too much focusing power for the length of the eye. If the cornea and the crystalline lens had less combined focusing power, or if the eye were shorter, then the light rays would be focused precisely onto the retina.

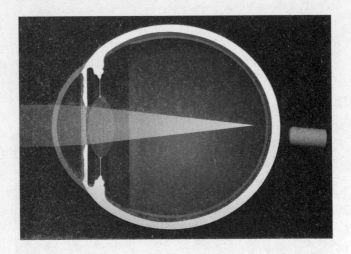

Nearsighted eye

Farsightedness. Farsighted people see faraway objects better than those that are near. Farsightedness (also known as hyperopia) results when the cornea and the crystalline lens together have too little focusing power for the length of the eye. Light rays from distant objects are focused not onto the retina but behind the retina. If the cornea and the crystalline lens had more combined focusing power, or if the eye were longer, then the light rays would be focused precisely onto the retina.

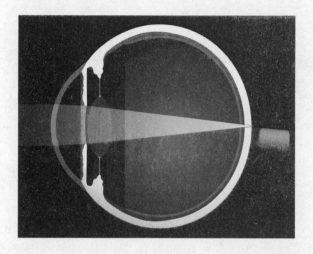

Farsighted eye

Astigmatism. People whose eyes focus light rays unevenly have astigmatism. Astigmatism occurs when the cornea has an irregular shape. The cornea should be round and symmetrical like a basketball, but in cases of astigmatism it is shaped more like a football. People with astigmatism see both near and far objects out of focus. Astigmatism frequently accompanies nearsightedness or farsightedness.

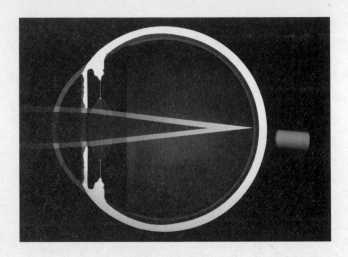

Astigmatic eye

Presbyopia. Presbyopia (which comes from the Greek for "old vision") refers to the gradual loss, as we age, of the eye's ability to adjust the focus from far to near. Presbyopia is a normal part of the aging process, affecting each and every person, and usually begins to cause a problem with near vision between the ages of forty and fifty. It is corrected by the use of reading glasses or bifocals.

Presbyopia occurs because the crystalline lens no longer adequately adjusts its shape to focus clearly on close-up objects.

Though presbyopia is referred to as "farsightedness" by many people, it should not be confused with true farsightedness (hyperopia). Presbyopia is caused by difficulty in changing the focus from far to up close—a problem with the crystalline lens. True farsightedness is caused by too little focusing power in the eye—a combi-

nation of the cornea and the crystalline lens. Both presbyopia and hyperopia cause blurring of the close-up vision, though hyperopia can blur the distance vision as
well. Whereas presbyopia is an aging effect and begins
to be experienced sometime after thirty-five years of
age, hyperopia affects people of all ages, even young
children.

Presbyopia can be present by itself or in combination
with nearsightedness, farsightedness, or astigmatism.

In ancient times, people with focusing errors had to
live with blurry vision. During the late Middle Ages
(around A.D. 1250), the first glasses were developed.
For almost seven hundred years, glasses were the only
treatment available for focusing errors. In the 1930s,
hard contact lenses were developed, followed in the
1970s by soft contacts.

Glasses and contact lenses improve vision by helping
the eye to focus the incoming light rays. They subtract
focusing power from nearsighted eyes and add focusing power to farsighted eyes. Bifocal lenses help
people with presbyopia to see faraway objects (through
the upper portion) as well as near objects (through the
lower portion).

||||||||||||||||||||||||||||||

HOW DOES
EXCIMER LASER SURGERY
IMPROVE VISION?

A laser is a device that creates a very special kind of light energy. The light can be of any color and can be invisible to the human eye.

The excimer laser makes pulses of invisible ultraviolet light. Each pulse of light removes a microscopically thin layer from the cornea, changing the curvature of the cornea ever so slightly. A computer running specialized software determines the exact pattern of pulses needed to remove the right amount of corneal tissue.

To correct nearsightedness, the curvature of the cornea must be decreased—the cornea must be made flatter. Tissue is removed in a disc-shaped pattern. To correct farsightedness, the central portion of the cornea must be made steeper. This is accomplished by removing tissue in a doughnut-shaped pattern. To correct astigmatism, the cornea must be made more symmetrical.

The excimer laser pulses may be applied to the surface of the cornea, using the technique known as PRK.

Alternatively, the excimer pulses may be applied to the cornea under a thin flap of tissue, using the technique known as LASIK.

Only a very small amount of tissue is removed, usually less than the thickness of a hair. Mild focusing problems will require small amounts of tissue removal.

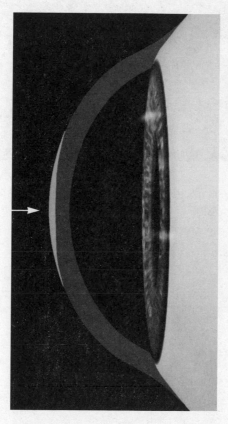

To correct nearsightedness, farsightedness, and astigmatism, the laser removes a small amount of tissue (see arrow) from the cornea, causing the shape of the cornea to change ever so slightly.

Severe focusing errors will require greater amounts of tissue removal. The total treatment usually takes less than one minute of actual laser time.

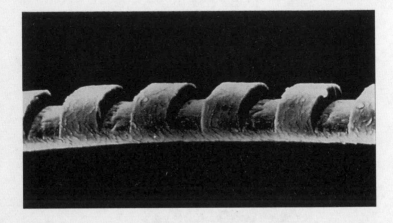

Excimer lasers are very precise! This is a human hair etched by an excimer laser.

ARE YOU
A GOOD CANDIDATE?

Some people should definitely not have excimer laser treatment. These include:

- People who are very happy wearing glasses or contact lenses. They have no need for the procedure.

- People under eighteen years old. Their focusing error is probably still increasing. But there is no upper age limit for excimer laser treatment.

- People whose vision is significantly changing. Glasses or contact lens prescriptions often continue to change through the teenage years into the early twenties. At least two years should pass without a significant change. (A significant change is one half diopter or more.)

- People who insist upon a perfect correction. A perfect correction is possible but cannot be guaranteed.

- Women who are pregnant or who are breast-feeding. Hormonal changes will often cause temporary changes in nearsightedness, farsightedness, or astigmatism.

You should consider this procedure, first of all, if you are not in any of the above categories. Second, you must have nearsightedness, farsightedness, or astigmatism. You may have presbyopia as well, but presbyopia cannot currently be corrected with the excimer laser, except through a technique known as monovision (see the chapter entitled "If You Are over Thirty-five," page 67). Third, you must want to be free of your glasses or contact lenses to the extent that you are willing to invest the time, energy, and money to understand and undergo the procedure. Even then, not everyone who wants to have the procedure will be able to, at least not now.

THE PRESURGICAL
CONSULTATION

The presurgical consultation is a very important part of the excimer laser surgery process. You can expect the following issues to be addressed during the presurgical consultation, and it is important that you are comfortable with the resolution of each issue.

Refraction. The doctor must determine whether you are a suitable candidate for the procedure. This depends on a variety of factors, including your age and occupation, but the doctor will be concerned primarily with your refractive (focusing) error—that is, your glasses or contact lens prescription. The doctor's recommendation to proceed or not will depend on an assessment of all the factors. An initial consultation may be scheduled to determine if you are a good candidate, with final measurements taken at a later consultation. If you wear soft lenses, you will need to stop wearing them at least one week before the final consultation; if you wear hard or gas-permeable lenses, stop wearing them at least six weeks before the final consultation. This is very important, because contact lenses can temporarily alter the shape of the cornea and the natural shape of your cornea must be accurately determined prior to the excimer procedure.

Complete Examination. Your doctor will perform a complete eye examination to determine the overall health of your eyes. Certain eye conditions may make you less suitable, or even ineligible, for the procedure. Included in this examination should be several tests, all of which are entirely painless, including a computer-assisted measurement of the contour of your cornea, known as corneal topography, a measurement of your pupil size in the dark, and a measurement of the thickness of your cornea. (For more details on these tests, read "Four Important Tests—and What They Mean," page 94.)

When Claire, a fifty-three-year-old photographer, had her topography done, she rested her chin on a metal bar and stared for a few seconds into a concave dome covered with concentric black and white lines similar to a target. She stared into the dome for a few seconds with one eye and then with the other. "You don't touch anything, and it doesn't touch you," Claire explained. A minute later, a computer on the other side of the dome printed out a topographical map of the shape of her cornea, showing how steep it was from point to point.

Doctor's Experience and Bedside Manner. You should meet the surgeon and make sure that you feel very comfortable with his or her education, bedside manner, and refractive surgery experience. Is the doctor board certified in ophthalmology? How long has the doctor been performing excimer laser surgery? How many LASIK or PRK procedures has he or she performed? How many procedures does the doctor perform each week? Does the doctor enjoy a good reputation in the community? You need to have complete confidence in the surgeon who will perform the procedure.

Pros, Cons, and Alternatives. The advantages, disadvantages, and alternatives to excimer laser surgery must be thoroughly discussed. What are the chances of actually achieving your desired results—good vision without glasses or contact lenses? Be sure to understand what problems might arise. And remember that nonsurgical treatments—glasses or contact lenses—always remain an option.

Informed Consent. You will be asked to sign papers confirming that you understand the risks and benefits of, and alternatives to, excimer laser surgery. These papers may contain words or ideas that you do not understand. Consider taking the papers home for slow, careful review before signing them. Also consider having a relative or friend review the papers to help you better understand them. Do not sign the papers until you completely understand all the words and concepts. These papers are legally binding and are designed to ensure that you understand the important aspects of the procedure. You do not have to sign the papers at the time of your initial consultation, although you cannot undergo the surgery until you do sign them.

Costs. All financial arrangements should be openly discussed. Often the fee can be paid by credit card, or your doctor may have a financing plan. Beware of fees that are unusually high or low. The fees for this procedure are not regulated in any way. Abnormally low fees raise questions of quality, and abnormally high fees may not be justified.

If you don't know anyone who has had excimer laser treatment, ask the doctor to put you in touch with a few patients. Stacy decided to have LASIK after a friend who had undergone the procedure described it to her in detail. The personal testimonial made all the difference. "She told me everything I would be feeling," Stacy said. "It really helps talking to someone who's had it done. A doctor can tell you the technical stuff, but hearing it from someone who's been through it is a lot different."

PRK OR LASIK?

The original form of excimer laser treatment is known as PRK (photorefractive keratectomy). In PRK, the laser energy is applied to the surface of the cornea, so no additional cutting of the cornea is required. The most popular variation of excimer laser treatment is called LASIK (laser in-situ keratomileusis). In LASIK, a thin flap of tissue is raised in the front of the cornea, and the laser treatment is then applied to the tissue beneath the flap.

When the laser treatment is applied to the tissue deep within the cornea instead of to the surface, the vision recovery is much quicker. Patients usually see quite well the day after LASIK, as opposed to waiting one or more weeks after PRK.

Neither PRK nor LASIK involves any pain during the procedure, but LASIK patients experience less post-treatment discomfort. In fact, many LASIK patients take no pain medicine after the procedure. PRK

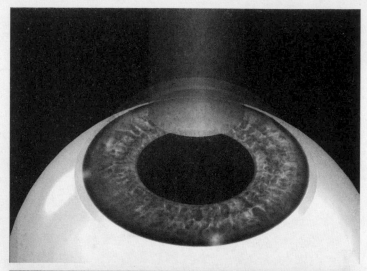

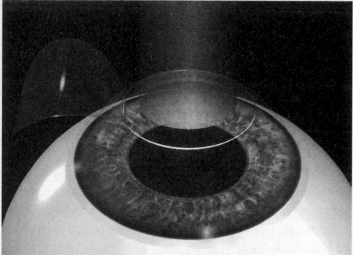

In PRK (top), the laser energy is applied to the surface of the cornea. In LASIK (bottom), a thin flap is made in the front of the cornea and the excimer laser treatment is then performed on the inner cornea.

patients will typically take pain medicine for a day or two. Most of the pain fibers in the cornea are in the surface portion. In PRK, the surface of the cornea is treated with the laser. In LASIK, the surface of the cornea is not treated, but is folded back so that the laser treatment is applied to the deeper tissue, resulting in very little post-treatment pain.

LASIK requires an additional surgical step, the creation of the flap. The flap is created with an instrument known as a keratome, which cuts and then folds back a thin layer of the front of the cornea. Creation of the flap takes about twenty seconds. During this time, most people have a feeling of "pressure" on the eye, though some people do feel slight pain. After the laser portion is complete, the flap is pushed back into its original position. No stitches are used, because the flap is held in position by natural corneal suction.

For most patients, the creation of the flap is the most worrisome aspect of excimer laser treatment. These flaps have been created for other eye procedures for over twenty-five years. Difficulties can occur with the flap, but in the hands of an experienced surgeon occur less than 1 percent of the time. Most of the complications with the flap are mild and can be easily treated. By far the most common problem is having the flap slide a little, causing wrinkles in the flap. When this occurs, it is most typically during the first day after the procedure, before the flap has had a chance to firmly set into position, and is corrected by lifting and repositioning the flap. Improper creation of the flap, resulting in either a partial or irregular flap, is the most serious complication and could conceivably lead to the need for further surgery or could prevent the doctor from performing the laser portion of the treatment.

Most people prefer the LASIK procedure because of the rapid vision recovery and minimal post-treatment pain. However, some people are not good candidates for LASIK, but are suitable for PRK. These would include people with very thin corneas, people with hobbies or occupations (such as boxing) where there is a good likelihood they will be hit in the eye, or people with specific, unusual conditions of the cornea. Although these patients might prefer to have LASIK, the PRK procedure would be a better choice. The decision of which technique is best in your situation must be made by you and your doctor.

THE SURGICAL EXPERIENCE:
THE PATIENT'S PERSPECTIVE

What is it like to have LASIK or PRK? Does it hurt? Is it frightening? Will it take a long time to recover? Do the benefits outweigh the risks?

Bruce, a forty-year-old accountant with 20/800 vision, was asking himself those questions as he sat in the waiting room on the morning of his surgery. He had been wearing glasses since the first grade. Without them, he was so nearsighted that he couldn't read the alarm clock from bed.

For years he had tried contact lenses, but he could never wear them for long. Within a few hours, wind and dust would leave his eyes red and teary. And he hated the hassle of caring for his lenses—the chemicals, the cleanings, the midnight runs to the drugstore for saline, and the constant worries about dropping a contact or having one get lost in his eye.

Glasses weren't much better. "I go swimming with

my children and take my glasses off, and I can't find my kids in the pool," he said. "I'm always fearful that I'll lose my glasses, and I won't be able to see. Peripheral vision is nonexistent, and for playing sports, that's important. I play basketball, ride my bike to work, horse around with the kids, coach the softball team. I don't want to overplay it, but in a certain way, it's a handicap."

Melanie, a twenty-six-year-old lobbyist, felt the same way. Like Bruce, she had been wearing corrective lenses since grammar school, switching back and forth between glasses and contacts. She had nearsightedness so severe, she said, that it left her "totally reliant on glasses or contact lenses for everything. If I knocked my glasses off my bedstand, I was helpless, crawling around on the floor trying to find them by feel. It drove me crazy. I felt so vulnerable."

Bruce decided to have PRK performed on his eyes. Melanie opted for LASIK. Before the procedure, they had complete eye exams. They read the eye chart, looked through different lenses, and had corneal topographies. Both were good candidates for laser eye surgery. They had healthy eyes, no illnesses, and no history of unusual scarring.

Still, as he sat in the waiting room, Bruce wondered if he was doing the right thing. "I'm a conservative, nerdy accountant watching my livelihood possibly going out the window. Not to mention seeing my family for the last time. The reality is that I'm probably more likely to get hit by a car riding home on my bike than I am to have something seriously go wrong with this procedure. You don't think about getting hit by a car when you ride your bike. But this is like, 'Okay, lie back, here it comes. Look at the red light.'"

Melanie had some preoperative jitters, too. "It was a little scary, because LASIK is a more invasive procedure than PRK," she said. "With PRK, there's no cutting of your eye and lifting it up. The cutting was probably the one thing that made me the most nervous. I worried about what would happen if the flap didn't get back on the right way."

About twenty minutes before the surgery, a nurse will administer a combination of anti-inflammatory and anesthetic drops into the patient's eyes. Both PRK and LASIK are performed with local anesthetic eye-drops. No medication—injected, intravenous, or oral—is needed, although doctors sometimes give patients Valium to calm their nerves. Melanie took a Valium while sitting in the waiting room. Her legs felt a little wobbly as she walked into the laser treatment room. By the time she had the procedure, her eyes were completely numb.

The setting for laser eye surgery is anything but surgical. Both Bruce and Melanie wore their street clothes. Other than a computer, some chairs, and the laser itself, which is about seven feet long, the room was empty. Before a PRK or LASIK patient enters the room, a technician programs the laser's computer to provide the exact set of excimer pulses needed to correct his or her refractive error.

Bruce sat in a reclining chair, similar to the kind

found in a dentist's office, and the doctor positioned him under the laser. The doctor put a U-shaped pillow around Bruce's head to keep him from moving and placed an eye patch over his left eye. He then put a small metal speculum, also known as a retractor, around Bruce's right eye to hold the eyelid open.

Up to this point, Melanie's experience was identical to Bruce's. She sat in the same chair with a pillow placed around her neck. The doctor covered one of her eyes and put a speculum around the eyelids of the other eye. Melanie had been dreading the speculum. "I suspected that it would be the worst part of the procedure and that it would hurt, but it wasn't really that noticeable. You could feel someone touching and moving your eyelid a little bit away from your eye, but there was no pain." Although Melanie couldn't close her eye, she could move it in any direction.

The primary differences between PRK and LASIK occur at the beginning and end of the surgery. For Bruce's PRK, the doctor put the speculum around Bruce's eyelid and then used a small metal instrument to wipe away the epithelium, the most superficial layer of his cornea. Bruce could see a shadow passing across his eye, but all he felt was a little bit of pressure. There wasn't any pain, and it took only a few seconds for the doctor to finish. Some doctors use the laser itself to remove the epithelium during PRK; others believe that manual or chemical removal is preferable.

For a LASIK patient like Melanie, the doctor needed to create a thin flap in the front of her cornea that could be peeled back to reveal the tissue underneath. Melanie stared at a small light overhead and saw a machine called a keratome moving slowly across her eye. The keratome made a humming noise as it worked. It took only a few seconds for the machine to make the flap and fold it back. "When the flap was actually being lifted up, it was blurry for a moment," Melanie recalled. "I remember thinking what a strange sensation it was, but none of it hurt."

The laser portion of the surgery is similar for PRK and LASIK patients. The doctor told Bruce to lie still, to focus on the red, blinking light, and to relax. "Crisscross apprehension with nervousness, with excitement, with fear of the unknown—that's what I was feeling," Bruce said. But the doctor talked Bruce through the surgery, explaining to him exactly what would happen at each stage. Bruce heard the laser make a series of loud clicking noises, akin to a bug zapper, and he caught a whiff of something that smelled like singed hair. He felt no pain, and less than sixty seconds later, the laser stopped firing.

Like Bruce, Melanie had less than a minute of laser time. She noticed that as the laser sequence progressed, the red light on which she was focusing changed. "At the beginning, I couldn't even pinpoint where the light was. It was just a blur. But as they used the laser, I could tell my vision was getting better. It was a little sharper."

After completing the laser treatment on Melanie's eye, the doctor flushed it out with water—a strange sensation, Melanie remembered, because she could see the water being sprayed across her eye and could feel it trickling down the side of her face but could not feel it on her anesthetized eye.

Once the laser sequence ends, PRK and LASIK patients have slightly different experiences. When Bruce's surgery was over, the doctor put some drops in his eye, including an antibiotic to prevent infection and an anti-inflammatory medication to minimize discomfort. He then placed a clear contact lens in Bruce's eye to protect the cornea and decrease pain. Bruce sat up and looked across the room. There was an assistant standing a few feet away and, despite the fact that the contact lens made his vision somewhat cloudy, Bruce could read the man's name tag. "A total sense of euphoria came over me," Bruce remembered. "I wasn't blind, and the bonus was that I could really see."

After the doctor finished lasering Melanie's eye, he put the corneal flap back in place. Melanie experienced a momentary blurriness as he repositioned the tissue. The doctor put some drops in her eye. Then she looked up at his assistants. "I remember seeing them right away. For about three feet out, I could see really well, whereas before I wouldn't have been able to recognize my mom. Past that, things looked a little blurry, as if someone had smeared Vaseline on my glasses."

Melanie walked into the waiting room. Her eyes were

watering badly, but she felt elated. "There was no discomfort. No pain at all. And my vision from about
three feet away was great—much better than I had ever
had. It was really amazing."

WHAT TO
EXPECT AFTER SURGERY

Recovery After PRK

No healing process takes place instantaneously, and healing after PRK or LASIK is no exception. For PRK patients, the initial healing phase lasts only a few days. Vision improvement is noticed after the first several days, although it can take a month or two for vision to stabilize and up to six months to achieve maximum vision.

Bruce's recovery after PRK was fairly typical. Immediately after the procedure, he received applications of three kinds of eyedrops: steroid drops to control healing, antibiotic drops to prevent infection, and anti-inflammatory drops to minimize discomfort. The drops needed to be used at regular intervals. He was also given pain pills to take as needed.

Bruce went home after the surgery and ate dinner. A few hours later, the anesthetic wore off, and he felt like he had a hair in his eye. It was uncomfortable but not bad enough to warrant painkillers. He watched TV and then went to sleep.

The next morning, Bruce went back to see the surgeon. The ride to the office was difficult. Bruce's eye was tearing and was light sensitive.

For the next two days, Bruce felt a scratchy sensation in his eye, and his eye watered. Three days after the surgery, the doctor removed Bruce's protective contact lens. Immediately, Bruce noticed a big improvement in his vision. His eye was still a bit watery, but Bruce was very excited by his improved vision.

The next morning, Bruce woke up with no pain, no tearing, and very good vision. "It was golden," he said. He played a game of catch with his son that morning and returned to work two days later. His computer screen looked fuzzy around the edges, but within a few days, it was crisp. For several weeks he noticed slight fluctuations in his vision. "Sometimes my vision was incredibly clear, and sometimes not, as if there were a film over my eyes. It's not that I couldn't see. It's that I couldn't see as well toward the end of the day and at night."

Today, more than a year after his surgery, Bruce's vision is stable and sharp. The halos and slight fluctuations in his vision cleared up within a few months, and the only lenses he wears are nonprescription sunglasses. "I can see the backs of the baseball jerseys from our seats now," he said. "I can go swimming with my kids. I can wrestle with them. I can snuggle with them. The results of the surgery exceeded my expectations, and I still can't believe it."

There's no way to predict how much pain a PRK patient will feel after the procedure or how long it will take for vision to stablize. Most patients complain of only mild discomfort, including tearing, swelling, light sensitivity, and sometimes a stinging or scratchy sensation. A few PRK patients—about two out of ten—experience more significant pain for a day or two after surgery.

If only one eye is treated at a time, a patient can depend on the uncorrected eye while the other eye is healing, so driving and working can resume within several days. People who have both eyes treated on the same day may not see well enough to drive for the first week, or sometimes longer. Depth perception, which requires clear vision in both eyes, will be worse than usual immediately after the surgery and will improve as the eye heals.

Claire, the fifty-three-year-old photographer, had a quick and easy recovery from PRK. Her eyes felt gritty when the anesthetic wore off, but there was no real pain. To avoid irritating her eyes, her doctor told her not to wear makeup for at least three to seven days following the surgery. Within twenty-four hours, her initial discomfort had disappeared. Before the surgery, her vision was worse than 20/400 in each eye. Now it's 20/25.

For Ethan, recovering from PRK was more difficult. The thirty-two-year-old actor had 20/800 vision in both eyes. He decided to have his right eye treated first. After surgery, his eye was "painful but not unbearable" for a couple of days. It was swollen, watery, light sensitive, and slightly red. For two weeks, his vision was blurry, but he could drive using his untreated eye.

A month and a half later, Ethan had his left eye treated. During the procedure, there was absolutely no discomfort, but a few hours later "there was a really strong burning sensation in my eye."

Ethan's ophthalmologist removed the protective contact lens, which he thought might be causing the problem, and put some numbing drops in Ethan's eye. Ethan tolerated the pain for two more days. A few months after the surgery, Ethan had 20/20 vision in the right eye and 20/25 in the left.

After PRK, patients typically use steroid drops in decreasing amounts for up to four months. The first month they commonly use the medication four times a day. Each month, the dosage is decreased. By the final month, most patients need only one drop a day. The eyedrops are critical, because they affect healing and can be adjusted by the doctor to suit a patient's healing pattern.

Lori, a forty-six-year-old special-events planner, learned the hard way how important it is to use the drops diligently. Before having PRK, she couldn't get out of bed without putting her glasses on. For the first two days after the surgery, her eyes were swollen, watery, and so light sensitive that she could open them only a crack. On her doctor's recommendation, she took painkillers every eight hours. She slept a lot, but felt no pain. Four days after the procedure, she saw well enough to drive herself to work.

Lori was happy with her vision, but as the months

wore on, she started having difficulty driving at night. Her right eye was somewhat undercorrected. "That could have partially been my fault," she said. "You have to use the steroid drops every eight hours. It's not the kind of thing I'm diligent about, because I didn't understand why I was supposed to do it. I thought I was doing it to keep my eyes moist. I didn't realize the drops were for keeping the correction." Lori had her right eye retreated, and now has 20/25 vision.

It usually takes several weeks for very good vision to return after PRK, though small changes—sometimes undetectable to the patient—will continue to occur for many months more. After full stabilization, the results will be permanent. Changes in your vision may still occur after the stabilization period, but these changes probably have nothing to do with PRK and would have occurred even without the surgery.

RECOVERY AFTER LASIK

LASIK patients usually heal much more quickly than people who have PRK, because the surface of the eye is not treated with the laser. The top layer, or epithelium, of the cornea contains most of the cornea's nerves. The epithelium is removed in PRK, but remains intact in LASIK. The epithelium is part of the flap that gets folded back into place after the LASIK treatment. As a result, these patients typically feel much less discomfort.

LASIK patients also recover good vision more quickly than PRK patients. In LASIK, the laser treatment is applied to tissue deep within the cornea instead of to its surface, shortening the recovery period. Be-

cause LASIK patients don't need to wait for the epithelium to grow back, they generally don't experience the
blurriness and light sensitivity that often accompany
the healing process in people who have had PRK.
Whereas PRK patients will usually use the protective
contact lens for three or four days, LASIK patients will
not use the protective contact lens at all, or will at most
use it for one or two days. Most LASIK patients see well
the day after surgery, though small changes will continue for several months. As a result, most LASIK patients prefer to have both eyes treated at the same time
or just several days apart.

Melanie had a textbook recovery from her LASIK
treatment. After the surgery, like PRK patients, she received antibiotic and steroid eyedrops, but she did not
have to wear protective contact lenses. She was given
Tylenol with codeine to take if necessary but never
needed it.

Her eyes were watering and stinging after the procedure, and she wanted to go home to rest in a dimly lit
place. A few hours later, she felt well and went out to
dinner. She could see clearly for a distance of about
three feet and was able to read the menu without a
problem. Everything beyond that was slightly blurry.

By the time Melanie had finished dinner, her eyes
felt slightly gritty, as if she had some dust in them. She
went home, took an aspirin, and slept through the
night. The next morning, she woke up and looked
straight at the ceiling. It was in sharp focus. "I remember thinking what a miracle it was that I could already see that well."

The grittiness that had bothered Melanie the night

before had already dissipated, and her biggest complaint was that her eyes periodically felt dry, a sensation that lasted for about a week. After seeing the doctor, who told her that her eyes were healing nicely, she spent the day visiting museums and that night went to the theater. She could see the stage without glasses and had no problems with halos, glare, or light sensitivity.

The following morning, Melanie noticed her vision was significantly sharper than the day before. Two days after her LASIK procedure, she was back at work and had no problems reading, driving, or using the computer. By the end of the week, she stopped using the eyedrops, as she had been instructed. Her vision was so crisp by that point that she didn't even notice the subtle improvements in her eyesight that gradually occurred over the next month.

Today, Melanie has 20/25 vision. She has noticed that it takes a few moments for her eyes to adjust when she walks from her brightly lit office into the underground parking garage. She did get mild distance glasses to sharpen her vision when driving at night in unfamiliar areas, but doesn't use them for any other tasks.

Not all LASIK patients experience as little postoperative discomfort as Melanie. Diane, a forty-five-year-old physician's assistant, was severely nearsighted. Immediately after the procedure, she looked out the clinic window at the cityscape in the distance. "I could see distances I never could see with glasses, and I started crying. I couldn't believe it. It was a moving experience."

When the anesthetic wore off, Diane felt like she was

having a bad contact lens day. Her eyes were burning, red, and gritty. She was also light sensitive and saw halos at night. For the most part, she felt discomfort, not pain, although it periodically hurt to blink. "It felt like I was blinking over sandpaper," she recalled. She took some Tylenol with codeine the night after her surgery and used some Advil the following day, but the discomfort disappeared quickly—within twelve hours.

Two days after the surgery, Diane's vision was 20/40, and she was driving without glasses. Her close-up vision, however, lagged behind her ability to see distances. For about six to eight weeks, she had a hard time finding a focal distance for reading. She bought two pairs of reading glasses at the drugstore—one with a weak prescription, the other somewhat stronger—and occasionally used a lighted magnifying glass to read the newspaper. It was frustrating, but two months later, she needed glasses only when reading small print or driving in the dark, and the halos she had been seeing around lights at night had completely disappeared.

Ted's recovery from LASIK was similar to Diane's. Before the surgery, the forty-eight-year-old teacher had severe nearsightedness and astigmatism. Immediately after the corneal flap was returned to its place, he could see faces and read large print.

That evening, he felt like he had an ill-fitting contact lens in his eye. He wasn't in pain, but he was uncomfortable. He also was light sensitive and saw halos.

The next day, he could see distances, but things weren't in sharp focus. "It was like having glasses or contacts and needing a prescription change. Things weren't crisp," he said. He was also having trouble reading, a problem that cleared up about two weeks later.

The halos around lights disappeared four months later. These days, he doesn't use glasses at all. "I think it's tremendous."

HOW WELL
WILL YOU SEE?

It is impossible to predict precisely how well any specific person will see after excimer laser treatment, but most patients will no longer need glasses or contact lenses for distance vision. After the initial treatment, about 95 percent of patients will have 20/40 or better vision without glasses; 20/40 vision is good enough to pass the driver's license vision test without glasses. About 75 percent will have 20/20 or better vision without glasses; 20/20 is considered "perfect" vision. Only about 5 percent of patients continue to need glasses all the time for distance vision after excimer laser treatment, and about 15 percent will use distance glasses occasionally, such as for driving.

For patients with mild nearsightedness, farsightedness, or astigmatism, the percentages are even better. Patients with severe focusing errors will have lower percentages of 20/20 or 20/40 vision. The general rule is:

A higher percentage of accurate results will be obtained in people who require less treatment.

Even those patients who still use glasses for distance vision after the procedure will see better without glasses and use thinner lenses than they did before. If needed, the results can often be further improved with a repeat excimer laser procedure. This is discussed in the chapter entitled "Retreatments."

These results are very impressive, but it is impossible to tell you exactly what your results will be. No guarantees can be made about the outcome of excimer laser treatment in any individual case, because each person responds in a slightly different way. If you will be satisfied only with "perfect" 20/20 vision without glasses

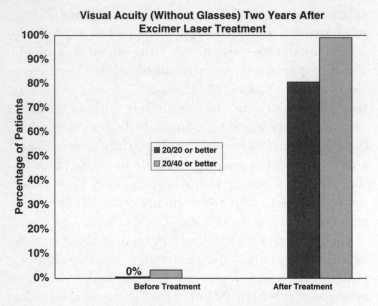

SOURCE: *"Apex Excimer Laser System Physician Information."*

after excimer laser surgery, then please do not have the surgery. Avoid any doctor or clinic that promises you a specific result, because that simply is not possible.

The quality of vision after excimer laser treatment may be superior or inferior to vision with contact lenses or glasses. Patients often have less glare than they had with contact lenses, and of course the inconvenience and discomfort of contact lenses is eliminated. Side vision isn't blocked, as it is with glasses, and there is no longer the problem of dirty, wet, or scratched glasses. However, while glasses and contact lenses can almost always provide 20/20 vision, this is not always possible with excimer laser treatment.

THE HEALING RESPONSE: THE
BIG VARIABLE

If eyes were made of marble, we could correct every one of them to a perfect 20/20. But eyes are made of living tissue. As can be expected, not all eyes display the same healing response. The individual healing response, which cannot be predicted accurately, affects the patient's final vision. Unfortunately, your eye's healing response cannot be predicted by how fast other parts of your body heal and cannot be determined by testing.

In LASIK, there is much less variation in the healing pattern of the eye. The healing pattern varies more when the surface of the eye is healing, as in PRK, than when the deeper tissue is healing, as in LASIK.

Most people exhibit a predictable healing pattern. As the eye heals during the first several weeks or months, there is a slight tendency for the eye to revert toward its initial state: nearsighted eyes will regress very mildly back toward nearsightedness and far-sighted eyes will regress slightly back toward farsighted-ness. Doctors take this tendency into account, and will create a small overcorrection initially. As a result, most patients will notice that their vision sharpens dur-ing the first several weeks or months of the healing period.

Some patients display a healing pattern known as re-gression, in which the eyes revert a greater amount than is normal. These people may have excellent vision during the early healing period, which then regresses into an undercorrection. Fortunately, undercorrec-tions are very easily improved with a retreatment.

Extensive exposure to ultraviolet light, such as from the sun or from tanning salons, during the first six months after treatment may cause some patients to un-dergo regression. It is very important for patients to protect their eyes from excessive amounts of ultra-violet light by wearing sunglasses when in the sun dur-ing the first six months after treatment, though small amounts of sun exposure will not be detrimental. Skiing, high-altitude sports, water sports, and beachgoing involve a great deal of ultraviolet exposure, so it is particularly important to protect your eyes by wearing sunglasses during these activities. Excessive ultraviolet light is also harmful to other parts of the eye (it can cause cataracts and damage the retina), so it is wise for everyone, whether or not they have recently had excimer laser treatment, to protect their eyes from the harmful ef-fects of the sun.

Everyone heals differently, and the differences can

significantly affect your final result. This is one of the reasons why it is so important to pick your doctor carefully. Regardless of the accuracy of the laser, it is still the doctor who uses the laser and then manages your healing response afterward. Be sure you understand your postoperative instructions, so that you will do everything you can to help with your final result.

||||||||||||||||||||||||||||

COMPLICATIONS:
WHAT CAN GO WRONG?

Excimer laser treatment is subject to complications, but the complication rate is very low. Patients often ask if one of these complications is likely to occur to them. It is impossible to predict whether a complication will occur in any specific case. Complications are rare but will be more common in people with high amounts of nearsightedness, farsightedness, or astigmatism, because these people require larger amounts of treatment. Most complications can be partially or totally corrected through a repeat laser procedure.

Patients commonly ask if they can go blind from the excimer procedure. No person has ever gone blind in any of the extensive FDA studies, but it is remotely possible. A severe infection, severe haze formation that did not respond to treatment, or a severe problem with the flap formation could result in greatly decreased vision, though further excimer laser treatment or other surgery would restore vision in almost every one of these cases.

During the first few months of healing, it is common for patients to experience difficulty with vision, including blurred vision, double vision, halos, glare, and light sensitivity. A foreign-body sensation and excess tearing will also occur in many people during the first month of healing. These symptoms are generally temporary and are a normal part of the healing process. Some people will experience difficulties that persist longer than one month.

The most common problems of laser vision correction include undercorrection and overcorrection, optical aberrations, dry eyes, infection, flap problems, and decrease in best-corrected vision.

UNDERCORRECTION OR OVERCORRECTION

By far the most common complication of excimer laser treatment is undercorrection or overcorrection. These complications occur because the patient experiences an abnormal healing response or because the laser energy removed slightly too much or too little tissue.

In the case of an undercorrection, the patient will be left with some degree of the initial focusing problem, though much less so than before. Further laser treatment, known as an "enhancement" or a "touch-up," can then be used to further improve the vision.

An overcorrection will result in a reversal of the vision focusing error: an overcorrection of nearsightedness will result in farsightedness, and vice versa. In most cases, an enhancement laser treatment can be performed to improve the resulting focusing error.

Undercorrections and overcorrections are the main

reason that all patients do not have perfect 20/20 vision after the excimer laser treatment. No patient can be guaranteed perfect vision after excimer laser treatment. If you will be satisfied only with 20/20 vision, then you should not have the procedure, because this result cannot be guaranteed.

OPTICAL ABERRATIONS

Optical aberrations are very common during the first six months of healing. During the first six months after laser vision correction surgery, 10 percent of patients reported glare and 10 percent reported halos around lights, though less than 1 percent described these problems as "moderate" or "marked." By the one-year visit, only 2 percent of patients reported these symptoms, and less than 0.5 percent reported the symptoms as "moderate" or "marked" (a). Ghost images may also occur, particularly during the early healing phases.

Retreatment may resolve problems with halos, glare, or ghost images, although many patients don't find these optical aberrations unduly annoying. For several weeks after having PRK, Bruce saw starbursts or halos around stoplights when he drove home at night. "It happens less and less," he said. "When it's pitch-black and there's only one light, that's when I get the starburst. When there are multiple sources of light, there are no starbursts at all." The starbursts disappeared a few months after surgery.

Optical aberrations most often occur if light is entering from around the edge of the treatment area. Some people have pupils that dilate in the dark larger than the treatment area. In these people, light passing around the treatment area may cause halos or glare at night. It is important that your doctor measures the size of your pupils in the dark. Newer lasers allow dramatically larger treatment areas with much less chance of glare or halos. If you have large pupils or large amounts of astigmatism (which in some lasers require the treatment zone to be made smaller), make sure that your procedure will involve an appropriately large treatment area.

Irregularity of the treated area, referred to as irregular astigmatism, may also cause optical aberrations. As the eye heals, the initial unevenness will significantly smooth out, causing the aberrations to improve significantly or completely disappear.

DRY EYES

Many people experience increased dryness of the eyes during the first few days or weeks of the healing period after laser vision correction. For most people, the feeling of dryness and irritation is merely a minor inconvenience and is treated by using moisturizing eye drops.

Dryness is more common in patients who have dry eyes before laser vision correction or who live in very dry environments. It is more troublesome during the winter months, when the humidity is lower. Dryness will cause irritation of the eyes and may cause a temporary decrease in the sharpness of the vision.

Melanie's dryness after LASIK was fairly typical: "My eyes felt a little scratchy for about a week. Nothing drastic, just something I noticed. It felt better when I put in the wetting drops. But after a week or so, I found that I didn't need the wetting drops anymore." However, some people experience extreme dryness after laser vision correction, which in very rare cases can last for many months.

If you are bothered by dryness after laser vision correction, you will need to use moisturizing drops. Air blowing across the face will dry out the eyes, so avoid wind, air conditioners, or open car windows. Often a humidifier in the bedroom or thicker drops at bedtime will also be very useful. In the rare case of prolonged dryness, special anti-inflammatory drops are usually very effective.

INFECTION

Just as with surgery on any part of the body, the eye is susceptible to infection during the early healing period after laser vision correction. You will be asked to follow certain instructions, including using antibiotic eyedrops and keeping water and makeup away from the eyes, during the first few days after your procedure. Carefully following these instructions will decrease the infection rate to much less than 1 percent. Even if an infection were to occur, use of antibiotic eyedrops should control the infection.

FLAP PROBLEMS

Creation of the protective corneal flap is the part of the LASIK procedure that most worries patients. In fact, in the hands of a skilled and experienced surgeon, flap problems occur less than 1 percent of the time and are usually minor in nature. The main flap problem is sliding and wrinkling of the flap, which most commonly occurs during the first day after the procedure, before the flap has healed solidly in place. This can occur by accidentally touching the flap with your finger or medicine dropper, or if the eye becomes very dry and the flap adheres to the eyelid. Movement of the flap will cause blurry vision, so your doctor will need to adjust the flap, which is painless and requires just a few minutes.

In very rare situations, the flap creation will not be optimal. When this occurs, the doctor will usually not proceed with the laser portion of the treatment. Instead, the doctor will ask you to wait several months for the flap to heal firmly. The doctor will then make a new flap and perform the laser treatment.

DECREASE IN BEST SPECTACLE-CORRECTED VISION

Best spectacle-corrected vision is the best vision obtainable when wearing the optimal pair of glasses. It is a measure of the best vision possible with glasses. Of course, you probably will no longer use glasses or contact lenses for distance vision after the surgery, so you may not even be aware if your best possible vision is slightly different.

For the majority of people, a mild decrease in best corrected vision is usually not noticed. A moderate loss of best corrected visual acuity would be noticed by every patient and might make it hard to work in occupations that require fine vision. Severe loss of best corrected visual acuity is exceedingly rare and in fact has not occurred in any of the FDA-sponsored tests.

Some professionals, such as commercial airplane pilots, care very much about their best corrected vision. These pilots must have best corrected vision of 20/20 in both eyes to maintain their licenses, so they should carefully consider the small risk of less than 20/20 best corrected vision.

In LASIK, unevenness of the flap, or in the tissue beneath the flap, could result in some decrease in best corrected vision. Small irregularities smooth out during the initial three months after the procedure, resulting in a gradual but noticeable improvement in vision. In one large LASIK study, 1 percent of LASIK patients experienced some decrease in best spectacle-corrected vision during the first three months. This decreased to 0.6 percent by the end of the first year (c). In another large laser vision correction study, 1 percent of patients had a decrease in best spectacle-corrected vision after one year, but every single patient in the study achieved 20/20 best-spectacle corrected vision (b).

||||||||||||||||||||||||||||

RETREATMENTS

Not all patients get a satisfactory result from excimer laser treatment. This may be due to undercorrection, overcorrection, or one of the complications described previously. By far the most common problem is an undercorrection or overcorrection.

Patients who experience undercorrection or overcorrection can usually undergo a second procedure, known as an enhancement, to obtain a better correction. In most cases, a significant improvement in the vision will occur, but it is important to realize that this, too, is a laser procedure and therefore has the same risks of the first laser procedure. It is possible but rare that your vision can be worse after an enhancement procedure. Complications can occur, even if no complications occurred during your first procedure.

If your vision is quite good after your excimer laser treatment, but not perfect, you should consider carefully whether you want to have an enhancement procedure. Maybe you can easily adapt by wearing glasses on a limited basis, such as for driving or watching movies. If your vision is really not satisfactory, then an enhancement procedure is a good idea.

Overall, around 10 to 20 percent of patients undergo enhancement procedures, though your likelihood will vary significantly depending on your degree of near-sightedness, farsightedness, and astigmatism. Over 25 percent of patients with extremely high degrees of nearsightedness, farsightedness, and astigmatism are likely to require enhancement procedures.

Lori ended up slightly undercorrected in both eyes after having PRK, which meant she was still somewhat nearsighted. She had excellent vision for close-up work, but distances were a problem—especially when driving at night. She got prescription glasses as a "security blanket," she said, "because it's a little scary to wait until you get right up to the street signs" to read them. But she decided soon after to have an enhancement procedure on her right eye.

The enhancement, Lori said, "was a snap, because I knew what was going to happen. It was like seeing a movie the second time." The procedure was identical to Lori's first surgery, except it took even less time to complete. She took a pain pill for less than twenty-four hours and never experienced any pain, swelling, or light sensitivity. "Having one eye done was a breeze, because I could rely on the other eye. It was like it didn't happen," she said. Within three days, she was driving without glasses, wearing makeup, and was back at work.

Ted decided to have touch-up surgery four months after he first had LASIK. He was 20/40 in one eye and

20/70 in the other, and was straining to see distances when driving.

The touch-up LASIK procedure differed slightly from the first operation. Rather than using the keratome machine to cut a thin flap in the cornea, the doctor was able to see the outline of the original flap and reopen it by hand. The procedure itself was painless, but Ted experienced slightly more postoperative discomfort after the second surgery than he had felt after the first. The corneal flap irritated his eyelid. "It felt like something was in my eye, and I wanted to rub it," he says. The doctor put in a protective contact lens, and the pain disappeared.

The next day, Ted could read license plates. His vision had improved to 20/25, and he wasn't feeling any discomfort. Today, he doesn't need glasses for reading or distance.

ONE EYE OR TWO?

As a patient you must decide: Do you want both eyes treated on the same day, or each eye on a different day? Each approach has advantages and disadvantages. Your decision may also depend on whether you are having PRK or LASIK.

When one eye is treated at a time, you can resume normal activities within a few days, because you can see well out of the untreated eye while the treated eye is healing.

Ethan had his eyes treated on different days. After the first PRK procedure, his vision was so blurry that he could barely see out of the treated eye. While it was healing, he wore a contact lens in the untreated eye. He could drive, read, and go to work. "I would just concentrate on seeing out of the one eye," he said. "It's difficult, but you can do it."

Nicole, a thirty-seven-year-old actress, also had PRK performed on her eyes on separate occasions. After her first surgery, her eye was tearing and scratchy. "It felt like someone had kicked a whole pile of sand into my eyeball," she said. She relied on painkillers to dull the discomfort and slept a lot during the next two days.

For the first month or two after the operation, Nicole wore a contact lens in the untreated eye. Her naturally dry eyes, however, caused the eye with the contact lens to become red and gritty. After a few weeks, Nicole decided to leave the lens out. "I just relied on my one good eye until the second eye was treated," she said. "That was fine."

Nicole's second surgery was easy in comparison to the first. She experienced less pain afterward and felt like "more of an old pro," she explained. "I covered the newly treated eye and read with my one good eye."

Treating one eye at a time is less convenient for many people, but it is definitely safer. The results from the first eye can be assessed and, if needed, alterations can then be made in the technique planned for the second eye. For example, if an overcorrection occurred in the first eye, less laser energy might be used for the second eye. It takes several months to know with certainty the final outcome from the first procedure. It is very common to have the second eye treated sooner than this, but patients need to know that their first eye is still undergoing some change for several months.

If both eyes are treated on the same day, then the healing for both eyes will occur at the same time. You will not have to go through two separate healing periods or a period of misbalance between the first and second eye treatments. However, your vision will be limited in both eyes at the same time as they simultaneously heal.

LASIK patients usually experience a rapid return of vision, so many LASIK patients elect to have both eyes treated on the same day. Most, but not all, LASIK patients who have both eyes treated on the same day are able to drive and return to work the very next day.

After having a long conversation with his doctor, David decided to have LASIK on both eyes on the same day. He knew that it might take longer for him to be able to see clearly and return to his normal life, but he couldn't tolerate contact lenses and didn't want to have to wear his thick glasses lens on one eye and nothing on the other while recovering from the LASIK. "The perceived benefit to me seemed so much greater than the risk," he said. For two days after his surgery, David had difficulty seeing, but by the third day, he was in good shape. In his mind, the temporary inconvenience was worth the price.

HOW TO
CHOOSE A DOCTOR

If you think surgical correction of nearsightedness, far-sightedness, and/or astigmatism may be for you, the most important choice you will make is the doctor, even more important than deciding whether or not to have the procedure. A conscientious surgeon will help you decide whether excimer laser treatment is right for you by highlighting the pros and cons as they relate to your particular situation. The surgeon should discuss the advantages and disadvantages of PRK, LASIK, and nonlaser procedures to help you choose which technique is best for you. The surgeon will also perform the procedure.

The role of the doctor cannot be overemphasized. Some clinics would like you to think that the laser does all the work and that the surgeon is not very important. Remember—the laser is just a tool the surgeon uses to correct your vision and, like other tools, the way it is used makes all the difference. The laser does not decide what to do—the doctor does. The laser performs the task that it is programmed for, so the measurements and information given to the laser by the doctor are critical. Also, the laser will not be monitoring your progress or initiating adjustments after the procedure—the doctor will.

The surgeon will decide which equipment to use and will make sure that the equipment is properly maintained and calibrated.

Be wary of clinics that de-emphasize the surgeon, and make sure that you know your surgeon and feel comfortable with his or her manner, education, and experience. Select a doctor that you trust and who you think has good judgement.

Be wary also of slick advertisements. A good advertisement means nothing more than the clinic has a good advertising agency. It does not mean that the doctor is right for you.

Be careful about referrals from other eye doctors. Many eye doctors have financial arrangements with specific laser clinics or surgeons and the referring doctor will receive financial benefit if the procedure is performed by the suggested clinic or surgeon. Carefully question the referring eye doctor and the laser surgeon to be sure that you know the details of this financial arrangement and make sure that you feel confident with your choice.

Carefully check the credentials of the surgeon. See if the doctor is board certified in ophthalmology and make sure that you respect the doctor's education, training, and experience. Has the doctor just started performing surgery to treat nearsightedness, farsightedness, and astigmatism, or has the doctor been doing so for many years? How many LASIK or PRK procedures has the doctor performed and how many does he or she perform each week? Is LASIK (or PRK) a major part of the doctor's practice or just one of many parts? As a consumer, you need to be aware that there are quality differences among surgeons and among laser centers, and that these quality differences may impact upon your chances of complication and your final visual result.

Does the doctor listen to you, and does the doctor clearly answer all your questions? Does the doctor seem to care about you and your individual needs?

|||||||||||||||||||||||||||||||

IF YOU ARE
OVER THIRTY-FIVE

If you are over thirty-five years old, please read this section very carefully. It may seem confusing at first, but it is very important that you understand it.

As people approach forty to forty-five, they begin to lose the ability to change their visual focus from far to near. When their eyes are adjusted for distance, either with glasses, contact lenses, or with laser eye surgery, there is difficulty in seeing clearly up close.

If you don't wear glasses or contact lenses, you will begin to need reading glasses for clear close vision when you approach forty to forty-five years of age. If your eyesight with glasses or contact lenses is clear for distance vision, you will need to wear reading glasses or bifocal glasses for near vision. Alternatively, you will need to take off your distance glasses or contact lenses in order to see clearly up close, because you will be unable to see near objects clearly with your distance glasses on.

People often mistakenly refer to this condition as

"farsightedness," but, in fact, it is not farsightedness at all. True farsightedness (hyperopia) is an inherent lack of focusing power in the eye and is not caused by getting older. The medical term for the change that occurs with aging is "presbyopia," which comes from the Greek words meaning "old vision." (Unfortunately, there is no English word for this condition other than the awkward "presbyopia.") Everybody develops presbyopia.

If you are nearsighted, farsighted, or have astigmatism and are developing presbyopia, you will probably need bifocal or trifocal glasses. The upper lenses of the bifocals are for distance vision; the lower are for close-up vision. Some people prefer trifocals, in which there are three pairs of lenses—an upper pair for distance, a middle pair for middle distances (about three to six feet), and a bottom pair for objects one to three feet away. Bifocal contact lenses exist but generally do not provide extremely sharp vision.

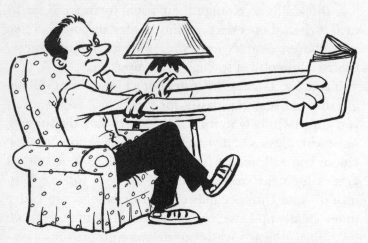

"Honey, I think my arms are getting too short!"

For those of you approaching or in this age group, you and your doctor must decide how best to correct your vision when you develop presbyopia. This decision must be made regardless of how you choose to correct your refractive error—either surgically or nonsurgically. People who have already begun to use bifocals, trifocals, or reading glasses understand this, but people who have not yet crossed this threshold or who simply remove their glasses when they read usually find this confusing.

You have three options to consider if you are nearsighted or farsighted and have presbyopia:

1. *Adjust for distance.* Both eyes can be fully adjusted for clear distance vision. But the patient will need to wear reading glasses for good close vision, usually beginning sometime between the ages of forty and fifty. This might be referred to as the "normal" situation, because most people start to need reading glasses at about that age.

Nicole, who is thirty-seven, decided to have both eyes adjusted for distance. A few months later, she started noticing subtle differences in her close-up vision. "It's not that I can't see up close," she explained, "but it's not as crystal sharp as it used to be. Threading a needle isn't as easy as it used to be. Before the surgery, I would take off my distance glasses to thread needles. I don't need reading glasses yet, but the perfect precision of close-up sight that I used to have is not quite there. I know it's just basically a part of getting older."

Claire, who is fifty-three, echoes those sentiments. She had both eyes corrected for clear distance vision, despite knowing that her close-up vision would not be as crisp after the surgery. She bought a pair of reading glasses at the pharmacy for $14. "I only wear them if I'm reading in bad light or reading tiny, tiny print," she said. "For someone my age, that's better than most of my colleagues."

2. *Monovision.* Monovision is when one eye is adjusted for distance vision and one eye for near vision. Monovision is often created with contact lenses for people over forty years old and can be created by any type of refractive surgery procedure. In monovision, one eye is primarily used at a time for ideal focus. The "distance" eye is primarily used to see far-off objects. The "close-up" eye is primarily used to see near objects. Both eyes are used all the time, but one is generally primary, depending on the distance of the viewed object. Peripheral vision is unaffected and depth perception is usually only mildly affected.

The main advantage of monovision is that patients often will not have to use glasses for distance vision or for near vision. The main disadvantage is that the patient is relying on one eye at a time, and some people do not like this. People with monovision may still use glasses in situations where they require excellent vision out of both eyes. Some, but not all, monovision patients will use glasses when driving a car (especially at night) or doing extensive reading. Other monovision patients will almost never use glasses.

Monovision is achieved by purposefully leaving one eye somewhat nearsighted when having laser eye surgery. Usually, this is the nondominant eye (often but not always the left eye in a right-handed person or the right eye in a left-handed person). If a patient chooses monovision and for some reason does not like it afterward, the "near" eye can usually be corrected for distance in a second laser procedure. This will eliminate the remaining nearsightedness.

Getting used to monovision generally takes several weeks but may take several months, because you are breaking very well established ways of using your eyes. People rarely ask to have monovision eliminated after they get adjusted to it.

Paul, a forty-three-year-old doctor, decided to have laser vision correction performed on his right eye. He improved his vision in that eye from 20/200 to 20/20, but he left his other eye uncorrected. He opted for monovision, he said, because "I'd like to be able to read without glasses. I'm also a microsurgeon. I like to be able to hold things very close to see them. If I had excimer on both eyes, I'd lose that ability very soon."

It took Paul about three weeks to mentally and physically adjust to monovision. Initially, he saw subtle halos in the dark, and his reading vision in the corrected eye was poor. He continued to wear a contact lens in his untreated eye for distance and didn't operate for three weeks after the surgery. Now, more than a year after his procedure, Paul doesn't require corrective lenses for any task. When reading and operating, he relies on his nearsighted eye. When he's driving or at the movies, his distance eye takes over.

3. *Mild monovision.* This is a compromise between full distance vision in each eye and full monovision. In

mild monovision, one eye is left with only a small amount of nearsightedness. This will cause only a small decrease in distance vision in that eye, but will aid somewhat in midrange and close-up vision.

For many patients forty-five or older, this mild monovision is a reasonable solution to the problem of nearsightedness, farsightedness, and astigmatism combined with the aging changes of loss of focusing. The degree of mild monovision is adjustable, based on the patient's age and visual demands.

Lori decided that, at the age of forty-six, mild monovision made more sense than a full correction for distance. After having laser vision correction, her vision improved to 20/25 in the right eye and 20/40 in the left. She doesn't need corrective lenses for reading or distance. "The joke among my friends is that I'm now the only one who doesn't need glasses," she said. "I love it."

There are only a few times during the day that Lori notices she has monovision—when she's putting on makeup or reading for long periods of time. When she looks up from a book, it takes a few seconds for her reading eye to readjust to see distances. And, she added, "When you're putting makeup on, if you close the eye that's corrected for close-up work, you're left with an eye that has distance vision and doesn't see as well up close. Other than that, you never notice."

Lori is thrilled with the results of her monovision. "It's freed me to see," she remarked. "I don't have to think about seeing, whereas when you wear glasses, you always think about seeing. You wake up in the middle of the night, and you can't go to the bathroom without a pair of glasses on. Now I go past the mirror in the middle of the night, and I'm startled because I think someone's in the room with me. Then I realize it's me. I've just never been able to see that far."

A small number of patients over forty with nearsightedness do not wear bifocal glasses, but merely take off their distance glasses when they want to read close-up. The key question you must ask yourself is: Can you read up close with your distance glasses on? If you *must* take off your distance glasses to read up close, then you have presbyopia. People with presbyopia who get both eyes fully corrected for distance vision will then need to use reading glasses to see clearly close-up. If you currently simply take off your glasses to read up close, then you should carefully consider whether or not you really want to have excimer laser surgery to eliminate completely your distance glasses prescription.

THE MOST
COMMONLY ASKED QUESTIONS
ABOUT EXCIMER LASER
TREATMENT

What are the odds of eliminating my need for distance glasses with excimer laser treatment?

Overall, 75 percent of patients will have perfect (20/20) vision without glasses, and 95 percent of patients will see well enough without glasses to pass the driver's license eye test (20/40). The results are better than this for patients with low amounts of correction and often can be improved by retreatment when needed.

Does excimer laser surgery hurt?

There is only mild discomfort during the procedure, usually less than having your teeth cleaned. For the first few days after LASIK, there is usually a mild scratchy sensation. PRK patients will experience a little longer and greater discomfort than LASIK patients.

Can I go blind from excimer laser surgery?

It is possible but very, very unlikely. No eye has ever had an extreme loss of vision in any of the FDA tests. A severe infection, uncontrollable haze after PRK, or an extreme problem with the flap formation after LASIK could cause significantly decreased vision. Even in this exceedingly rare possibility, the vision could usually be partially or completely restored by a repeat laser procedure or by other surgery, such as a corneal transplant.

What about the long-term results? Will my eyes deteriorate in the future?

Since 1988, several million LASIK and PRK procedures have been performed around the world. There is no evidence of anything that would adversely affect the long-term health of the eye. The keratome, a major part of the LASIK procedure, has been used since the 1970s without adverse long-term effects.

Which technique is better for me: LASIK or PRK?

Most doctors recommend LASIK over PRK for all of their patients, except in certain rare situations, due to the more rapid healing and virtual lack of pain. However, in your particular situation, PRK may be more appropriate. It is important to carefully consider the pros and cons of each technique.

What about other techniques to correct permanently nearsightedness, farsightedness, and astigmatism?

Several other nonlaser techniques now exist to correct permanently nearsightedness and/or astigmatism: radial keratotomy (RK), astigmatic keratotomy (AK) and the corneal ring (ICR or Intacs). Another laser technique, known as the holmium laser, is also capable of correcting farsightedness. Excimer laser surgery is superior to these other techniques in most situations, though these other techniques may be more appropriate in specific cases.

Will I need to wear an eye patch after the procedure?
No, though some people will need to wear a special contact lens for a few days.

I've heard that ultraviolet light can cause cancer. Can this laser cause cancer?
The excimer laser has been very carefully studied in this regard, and there is no risk of cancer from LASIK or PRK.

Will I be able to see anything during the procedure?
Yes. During the procedure, you will be asked to look at a blinking light. This will help to maintain proper alignment of the eye during the procedure.

What if I move during the procedure?
Patients worry about this a great deal, and their fear is largely unnecessary. Patients frequently move during the procedure. The doctor can stop the procedure at any time and resume when the patient is ready.

What if I blink during the procedure?
Your eye will be held open by a device known as a speculum, which usually doesn't hurt. You will not be able to blink.

Will scars form from the procedure?
In LASIK, there are only extremely faint scars that cannot be seen except with a microscope. In PRK, very faint, microscopic scarring (haze) is sometimes present after the treatment. Unless the haze is severe, it will not have any effect on vision.

Will excimer laser treatment cause cataracts or influence the later treatment of cataracts?

Excimer laser surgery is not known to cause cataracts and does not affect the removal of cataracts. However, if you know you will need cataract surgery in the near future, there is no need to undergo an excimer laser procedure; your nearsightedness, farsightedness, or astigmatism can be corrected as a part of the cataract implant surgery.

Will there be any limitations on my activities after excimer laser treatment?

There are no limitations on your activities, except that you will be asked to avoid getting water into your eye during the first week or so. Of course, you should not resume activities such as driving until your vision is adequate.

If I don't get a perfect 20/20 correction, will I be able to wear contacts after excimer laser treatment?

Some patients do not get a full correction with excimer laser surgery and will want to wear contact lenses. The general rule is: If you could wear contact lenses before the procedure, then you should be able to wear them afterward. If you were unable to wear contacts before the procedure, then you probably will not be able to wear them afterward. There are some exceptions to this rule. After surgery the cornea has a slightly different shape, so some patients who could wear contacts before the procedure will not find an adequate fit after. However, because there are so many contacts now available, this would be exceedingly rare. More often, the opposite is true: Some patients who could not tolerate the thick lenses that were necessary before the excimer procedure can wear thin contacts after the procedure.

If I don't get a perfect 20/20 correction, will I be able to have a repeat procedure to improve the results?

In most but not all cases a "touch-up" or "enhancement" procedure can be performed to improve the vision, often to 20/20.

My distance vision has recently been getting worse. Will laser eye surgery stop the eyes from getting worse?

No. Laser eye surgery can correct nearsightedness, farsightedness, or astigmatism that is currently present, but cannot stop this naturally occurring condition from developing in the future. If your distance vision is significantly changing, you may want to delay the procedure until your distance vision stabilizes. In most people, distance vision stabilizes during the early twenties, though significant changes can occur at other times.

What are the most common negative side effects of excimer laser treatment?

Undercorrection or overcorrection are the most common negative results of excimer laser treatment. Usually this can be corrected with a second, "touch-up" procedure. Glare or halos are common during the healing period but almost always resolve over time.

I am very nervous about the procedure. Is this normal? Can I take Valium before the procedure?

Everyone is nervous about having a procedure performed on his or her eyes. This is normal human nature. Some doctors will give you relaxation medication prior to the procedure, but it is important to take only medication prescribed by your doctor.

PART II

||||||||||||||||||||||||||||

ADDITIONAL INFORMATION

—

FOR THOSE WHO WANT TO KNOW MORE

WHAT
DOES "20/20" MEAN?

The most important aspect of vision is known as "acuity," the ability of the eye to distinguish fine details. Acuity is measured by the smallest letters the patient can see on an eye chart. In the United States, we use twenty feet as a standard testing distance, and so "20" is always used as the first number in the visual-acuity measurement.

The second number in the measurement refers to the size of the smallest letters the patient can see. Size 20 letters are the smallest letters that most people with "perfect" vision can see at the standard twenty-foot testing distance. Size 40 letters are twice as big, and size 200 letters are ten times as big. Thus, a patient with 20/40 vision, when tested at 20 feet, can see down to the size 40 letters, but cannot see letters smaller than that.

Each eye is measured separately and has its own acuity. There are actually three different measurements of acuity for each eye: visual acuity without glasses (known as "uncorrected" vision), visual acuity with the current glasses (which may not be very accurate!), and visual acuity with the perfect glasses (also known as "best spectacle-corrected visual acuity"). So a nearsighted person might have 20/200 vision without glasses, 20/30 vision with the current glasses, and 20/20 vision with the best possible glasses.

Normally we consider 20/20 to be "perfect" vision, although a small percentage of people (about 10 percent) have even better vision—20/15. People with 20/25 or 20/30 uncorrected vision have very good, but not perfect, distance vision. Although their friends may be able to read smaller letters than they can at a distance, these people will probably get by fine without

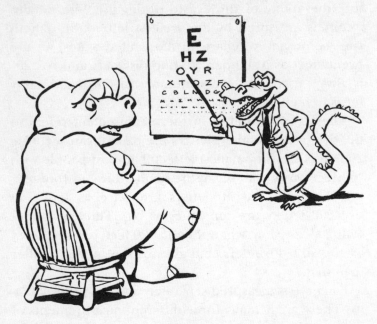

glasses for distance vision or may use glasses on a very limited basis, such as for driving or watching movies.

Most patients with 20/40 or 20/50 uncorrected vision use glasses for some things but not for everything. The patient will wear glasses to drive but might not wear glasses around the house. He or she would probably feel comfortable swimming or playing most sports without glasses. However, this is highly individual; some patients with this vision will wear glasses almost all the time.

In most states, a person must see at least 20/40 to pass the driver's license vision test. People with uncorrected vision worse than 20/40 legally have to wear corrective lenses to drive.

Most people with uncorrected vision worse than 20/50 will use glasses for distance vision most of the time. However, people vary in this regard; some prefer blurry vision to wearing corrective lenses.

Do all people with uncorrected 20/20 acuity have the same vision? No, other aspects of vision are also important. Dim lighting, side lighting, and glare can affect some people's vision more than others. This is known as contrast sensitivity. Contrast sensitivity can be measured, but this test has not gained widespread popularity.

||||||||||||||||||||||||||||||||||||||||||||||||||||||||||||||||||

HOW TO READ A GLASSES PRESCRIPTION

+2.00 –1.25 @ 90. This is a glasses prescription for a patient with farsightedness and astigmatism.

The first number (+2.00) is the amount of nearsightedness or farsightedness (a minus sign is for nearsightedness; a plus sign is for farsightedness). The second number (–1.25) is the amount of astigmatism, while the third number (@ 90) is the direction (axis) of the astigmatism. If there is no astigmatism, the prescription will have only one number, in this example +2.00.

Glasses prescriptions are in diopters, which measure how strongly the lenses bend the light rays. This should not be confused with visual acuity measurements! For example, a 2.00 lens does not mean that the eye sees 20/200; however, the higher the diopter number of your glasses, the worse your uncorrected visual acuity will be.

||||||||||||||||||||||||||||||||||||||||||||||||||||||||||||||||||

HOW TO READ A CONTACT LENS PRESCRIPTION

+1.75 –1.25 @ 90 / 8.6 / 13.8

Your contact lens prescription will be slightly different from your glasses prescription. The first set of numbers will be the nearsightedness or farsightedness and astigmatism, but these numbers will vary slightly from your glasses prescription. Also, the contact lens prescription will include the curvature, size, manufacturer, and model of the contact lens. In the above example, 8.6 refers to the curvature of the lens and 13.8 is the size.

WHAT IS A LASER?
WHAT IS
AN EXCIMER LASER?

A laser is a machine that produces a special type of light that can be very accurately focused. Unlike the light produced by ordinary lightbulbs, laser light is both uniform and coherent. "Uniform" means that each light ray is always one precise wavelength (energy), whereas ordinary light is a mixture of many different wavelengths. "Coherent" means that the light rays are highly synchronized in space and time. Because of these qualities, laser light can be very intense and can be focused very precisely, making laser light useful in medicine and industry.

Different lasers produce light of different wavelengths. Some lasers produce light that is visible to the human eye, whereas other lasers produce light that is invisible, such as ultraviolet or infrared light.

The term "laser" is short for "Light Amplification by Stimulated Emission of Radiation," the process by which a laser produces its light. Some people become alarmed when they hear the word "radiation," because they know that some types of radiation (such as X rays) can cause cancer. All types of light, including the normal light that we see, are a form of radiation. You do not have to be concerned: Eye lasers use light, but these lasers do not cause cancer.

The excimer laser used in eye surgery uses argon and fluorine gases to produce a beam of invisible, ultraviolet light. The laser light is then focused by a series of lenses, bounced off a series of mirrors, and mixed to create a more even beam pattern. Excimer lasers are very complex devices that can cost hundreds of thousands of dollars. In spite of the cost, excimer lasers have found a wide variety of uses in industry, ranging from glass etching to the sterilization of wines. The excimer laser can precisely remove tissue without causing scarring, which makes it ideal for reshaping the cornea.

Albert Einstein first proposed the principle behind the laser in 1916, but it was not until July 1960 that the

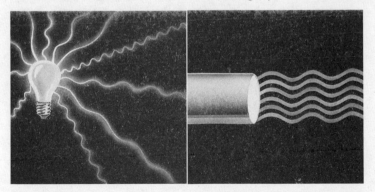

Ordinary light rays (left) are uneven. Laser light rays (right) are highly synchronized in space and time, and are one precise wavelength.

first laser was built. While most people are unaware of it, lasers are almost everywhere. Compact disc players use a laser beam to read the information encoded on the compact disc (which can be music, movies, or computer data). Lasers are also used extensively in communications, the military, and manufacturing, as well as in science. For example, a laser beam has been bounced off the moon and has measured the distance from the earth to the moon to within one inch.

Lasers are used in many fields of medicine, and their uses are increasing. Lasers can be used to remove wrinkles from the skin as well as polyps from the vocal cords. Orthopedic surgeons use lasers to remove tissue from inside damaged joints, and neurosurgeons use them to cut tumors off the spinal cord.

Lasers are used more often in ophthalmology than in any other field of medicine. In ophthalmology, lasers have been used for over thirty years and are used on a routine basis. In 1963, just three years after the invention of the laser, one was first used to treat a diseased eye.

Lasers are used to treat several different types of eye problems, and several different kinds of lasers are used. Argon lasers are used to treat complications of diabetes within the eye, as well as to lower the pressure inside the eye in cases of glaucoma. Krypton lasers are used to seal off dangerous new blood vessels that can grow under the retina. YAG (yttrium-aluminum-garnet) lasers are used to vaporize cloudy membranes that can form inside the eye after cataract surgery. Hundreds of thousands of patients undergo these different laser procedures every year.

THE HISTORY
OF THE EXCIMER LASER

An "excimer," short for "excited dimer," is a molecule that exists for only a fraction of a second, emitting ultraviolet light as it disintegrates. This light is then harnessed into a laser. Excimer laser technology was originally developed at IBM in 1976 with the hope that it would be useful for etching computer chips.

In late 1982 and early 1983, R. Srinivasan, Ph.D., an IBM researcher in Yorktown, New York, was testing the excimer laser to etch different materials. He described the exquisite manner in which the excimer laser could etch plastic without causing associated heat damage to the neighboring material. He also showed the effects on biological material, such as bone, cartilage, and hair. Dr. Srinivasan demonstrated that smooth grooves could be reproducibly etched into a human hair without burning or otherwise damaging the surrounding portions of the hair strand.

Stephen Trokel, M.D., an ophthalmologist at

Columbia University in New York City, saw a picture of the etched hair and visited Dr. Srinivasan at his IBM laboratory in July 1983. There, Dr. Trokel performed laboratory studies and confirmed that a very important technological breakthrough had occurred. From that point on, much research and development began to occur all over the world, most extensively in the United States.

The first excimer laser surgery was performed in 1985 by Dr. Theo Seiler of Germany, who used the laser to make an incision in the cornea, similar to the incisions made in radial keratotomy. Animal tests quickly confirmed that the excimer laser could more optimally reshape the cornea by removing a thin layer of tissue from the cornea's surface, a technique known as "photorefractive keratectomy" (PRK).

In February 1987, Francis L'Esperance, M.D., of Columbia University became the first doctor to use the excimer laser on a human being for PRK. One of the first patients had cancer inside his eye and was going to have the eye removed. The patient agreed to allow his eye to undergo this experimental treatment before it was removed. In 1988, the first normally sighted eye underwent PRK for the correction of myopia. This was performed by Marguerite McDonald, M.D., at Louisiana State University.

The LASIK variation was first performed on a blind human eye in 1989 by Ioannis Pallikaris, M.D., in Keraklion, Crete, who began performing the technique on sighted eyes in 1991. LASIK was first performed in the United States in 1991.

Testing the excimer laser as a treatment for nearsightedness quickly spread around the world. Many important refinements in the techniques occurred, resulting in improved results. As the high degree of safety and effectiveness became apparent, doctors in many countries began using the excimer laser. Modifications allowed the laser to treat astigmatism and farsightedness as well. During the late 1990s LASIK gained enormous popularity and became the predominant variation of excimer laser treatment. Exact figures are not available, but it is estimated that several million excimer laser treatments have been performed. Today, excimer laser treatment (predominantly LASIK) is being performed in every advanced country of the world.

WHO MONITORS
THIS TECHNIQUE?:
THE ROLE OF THE FDA

The Food and Drug Administration (FDA) is the agency of the U.S. government responsible for ensuring that drugs and medical products are safe and effective. Each manufacturer's excimer laser must be approved as safe and effective by the FDA before it can be used routinely in the United States. Most countries around the world have similar agencies that investigate and monitor medical products, but none are as thorough and demanding as the FDA.

Before 1938, new drugs or medical devices could be used in the United States without any study or approval by the government. If significant complications occurred, then the federal government would investigate the product and, if necessary, remove the product from the market. The Food, Drug and Cosmetic Act of 1938 requires manufacturers to test drugs and medical products thoroughly before they sell them to the general public. Although this process significantly delays the introduction of new drugs or devices, it does prevent most dangerous products from reaching the marketplace.

How does the FDA decide whether a product is safe? First, the product is tested on animals, and if the results are favorable, carefully controlled human tests conducted in the United States will follow. Only small numbers of people are tested at first, and if the results are favorable, larger numbers of people are tested. The FDA approves a drug or product only if it is convinced that adequate numbers of people have been tested and that these tests have been carefully conducted and their results adequately studied.

In the case of excimer lasers, each manufacturer conducts large-scale FDA studies. As advances are made in laser design, each substantially different or improved device must first be tested under the auspices of the FDA. The original small-scale FDA studies were begun in 1988 and were performed on blind or partially sighted eyes. Large-scale testing involving several thousand patients began in 1991, and the mandatory two-year follow-up period ended in 1994. Currently, over ten companies are involved in FDA-supervised tests of refractive eye laser technology. At least six laser companies have completed the rigorous FDA tests and achieved FDA approval.

FOUR IMPORTANT
TESTS—AND WHAT
THEY MEAN

During the course of your presurgical evaluation, your doctor will perform tests on your eyes to assess your suitability for excimer laser treatment. These tests include corneal topography, low-light pupil size, corneal thickness, and refraction.

MAPPING THE CORNEA:
CORNEAL TOPOGRAPHY

Corneal topography is a fascinating technique that uses a computer and a video camera to create a detailed map of the surface of the cornea. Over five thousand individual points on the cornea are measured within a fraction of a second. The computer then generates a map of the entire cornea, using different shades to represent different curvatures. Subtle variations in the curvature of the cornea can be detected.

Corneal topography maps help the doctor to evalu-

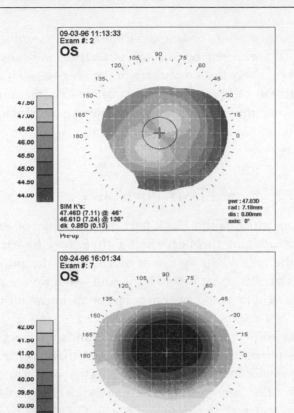

These cornea maps show the effects of the laser treatment. The computer map at the top was taken prior to the excimer laser procedure and shows an eye with moderate nearsightedness and astigmatism. Each shade of gray represents a different degree of curvature. The laser treatment alters the cornea curvature, as evidenced by the map at the bottom. These curvature changes are much too small to be appreciated without these sophisticated mapping techniques.

ate the cornea prior to laser treatment. For example, a map taken during the presurgical evaluation will sometimes reveal abnormal curvatures of the cornea, such as the condition of keratoconus, that make LASIK unadvisable. After the excimer laser treatment, your doctor will often use corneal topography to follow your course of healing.

Low-Light Pupil Size

The pupil, which is the black part in the center of the eye, is the opening through which light enters the back area of the eye. When we are in bright light, the pupil becomes smaller to let in less light, and when we are in a dark area, our pupil becomes larger to let in more light.

Just as some people have larger hands or necks, some people have pupils which are larger than average, particularly in low-light conditions. This may cause problems after laser vision correction, especially if the pupil gets much larger than the portion of the cornea treated with the laser. In such a situation, some of the light rays passing through the pupil will have passed through untreated portions of the cornea, and these light rays will not have the proper focus. When these light rays mix with the properly focused light rays, especially in low-light conditions, the result may be glare, halos around lights, or blurriness at night.

These difficulties with night vision can often be avoided by measurement of the pupil size in low-light conditions. People with extremely large pupils are at a greater risk of developing these side effects and should only have LASIK or PRK with a laser that produces appropriately large treatment areas. However, additional factors, such as very large corrections, also increase the likelihood of developing glary halos or blurriness at night.

Corneal Thickness

The cornea is composed of many layers of fibers, which combine to create the strength needed for the cornea to maintain its shape. In the LASIK procedure, a flap is made and tissue is then removed beneath the flap. It is important that enough tissue is left undisturbed to ensure structural integrity of the cornea.

Prior to performing LASIK, your doctor should measure the thickness of your cornea. This is performed with an ultrasound machine known as a pachymeter. Your doctor will then calculate whether your cornea is thick enough to perform LASIK. If you are not able to have LASIK because your cornea is not thick enough, you can usually have PRK. PRK does not involve making a flap and can usually be performed on corneas that are too thin for LASIK.

Refraction

A person has nearsightedness, farsightedness, or astigmatism because the light is not being focused accurately onto the retina at the back of the eye. The careful measurement of the exact correction needed for clear focusing is known as a "refraction." The refraction is the most important measurement, because it

determines exactly how much the cornea must be al-
tered to achieve excellent vision.

A refraction is performed through a technique of
trial and error by asking the patient to compare different lenses placed in front of the eye. Patients often
worry that they are giving inaccurate responses, but the
doctor will go over the same choices again and again to
ensure consistent responses.

In this high-tech field, the trial and error method of
refraction seems rather archaic. In fact, lasers can be
used to perform refractions, but no laser refractions to
date have proven to be more accurate than the "which
is better, one or two" method.

The refraction used for laser surgery must be performed with great care by a doctor skilled in this technique. Usually, as a double check, the refraction is
repeated after the eye has been dilated, in which the focusing muscles inside the eye have been temporarily inactivated. If there is any uncertainty about the
accuracy, the refraction can be repeated a third or
fourth time.

‖‖‖‖‖‖‖‖‖‖‖‖‖‖‖‖‖‖‖

ANOTHER USE
FOR THE EXCIMER LASER:
REMOVING CORNEAL SCARS

Although the correction of nearsightedness, farsightedness, and astigmatism is certainly the most common use of the excimer laser, this tool is also used to remove corneal scars. Thousands of people suffer from blindness caused by spots (called "opacities") in their corneas. Opacities can result from scarring after an injury or infection, or from hereditary diseases that cloud the cornea. If the cornea is not clear, it cannot transmit light rays. This results in worsened vision and, if severe enough, in total blindness. Thousands of corneal transplants are performed each year to treat cloudiness of the cornea.

Many patients can have their sight restored with the excimer laser, thus avoiding corneal transplant surgery. If the cloudiness is limited to the front portion of the cornea, it can often be removed by the excimer laser. This procedure is known as PTK (phototherapeutic keratectomy), and it requires less than one minute of laser application. The treatment itself, as well as the recovery, is similar to excimer laser PRK.

PTK represents a vast improvement over corneal transplants in terms of ease of treatment, complications, and cost. Unfortunately, the excimer laser can only remove opacities that are in the front 30 percent of the cornea or that are raised above the surface. Deeper opacities can be corrected only through a corneal transplant.

ALTERNATIVES
TO EXCIMER LASER
SURGERY

In addition to excimer laser treatment, several other techniques are currently available to treat near-sightedness, farsightedness, and astigmatism. All these treatments share the same goal as excimer laser treatment—to modify the focusing power of the eye in a predictable, safe, and permanent manner. Corneal rings and the holmium laser are currently used to correct focusing errors in selected situations. Implantable contact lenses look promising, but are still in the development and testing process. RK, AK, and ALK are now seldom used, having been replaced by more accurate techniques. Orthokeratology is a nonsurgical method to temporarily treat some focusing errors. And, of course, glasses and contact lenses are always available.

Corneal Rings (Intacs)

Corneal rings (also known as Intacs, intrastromal corneal rings, or ICRs) are small pieces of plastic that are embedded in the edge of the cornea. The arc-shaped rings make the central portion of the cornea flatter, decreasing the amount of nearsightedness. Currently, corneal rings are available to treat only low amounts of nearsightedness, and treatments for astigmatism and farsightedness are still being developed.

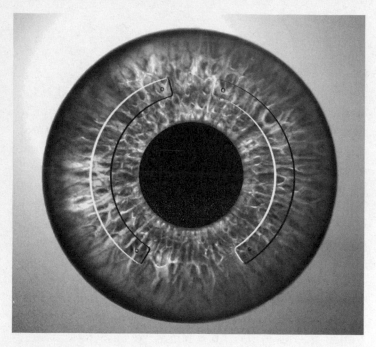

The corneal ring technique places two thin pieces of plastic in the edge of the cornea, which causes the central cornea to change shape.

By using rings of varying thickness, different amounts of nearsightedness can be corrected. However, corneal rings are made in only a limited number of thicknesses, so they can only be used for very specific corrections. If the visual result is not ideal, or if the eye changes in the future, the corneal rings can be removed, but there might not be another ring that is appropriate to correct your vision. In contrast, excimer laser treatments are available for a wide range of focusing errors and are easily adjustable with retreatments.

Holmium Lasers (LTK)

Farsightedness is the result of too little curvature of the cornea. In order to correct farsightedness, the central cornea must be made steeper. With the excimer laser, the central cornea is made steeper by removing tissue in a doughnut-shaped pattern from the peripheral cornea.

Another type of laser, known as the holmium laser, is also currently available to treat farsightedness. The holmium laser produces infrared light, which causes tissue to constrict, and is therefore very different from the ultraviolet excimer laser. The excimer laser reshapes the cornea by removing tissue; the holmium laser reshapes the cornea by causing tissue to constrict.

To treat farsightedness, the holmium laser is applied to the periphery of the cornea in a pattern of multiple spots. As this peripheral tissue constricts, the central cornea steepens, resulting in a decrease in farsightedness. This technique, known as LTK (laser thermal keratoplasty), takes only a few seconds and is effective in reducing lower amounts of farsightedness.

As with any other treatment, there is variability in how each individual responds. Currently, the holmium laser technique is limited to treating only small amounts of farsightedness and cannot treat astigmatism.

A similar technique, known as radio frequency keratoplasty (RFK) or conductive keratoplasty (CK), uses radio frequency energy to constrict the tissue. RFK is still in the development phase, but may someday also be available to correct farsightedness.

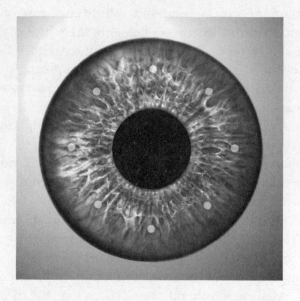

Holmium laser treatment for farsightedness (LTK). A series of focal treatments in the peripheral cornea causes the central cornea to steepen.

IMPLANTABLE CONTACT LENSES

Intraocular implants, also known as implantable contact lenses or phakic intraocular lenses, are tiny plastic lenses inserted inside the eye, behind the cornea. These lenses bend the incoming light rays and can correct nearsightedness, farsightedness, and astigmatism.

Intraocular implants have been used successfully for many years to replace the crystalline lens when it turns cloudy—forming a cataract—and has to be removed. When used to treat nearsightedness, farsightedness, or astigmatism, intraocular implants are placed in front of the crystalline lens, and the crystalline lens is left inside the eye. Some implants are placed in front of the iris (the colored part of the eye) and are known as anterior chamber implants. Others are placed behind the iris and are referred to as posterior chamber implants.

The long-term safety of intraocular implants for nearsightedness, farsightedness, and astigmatism has not been determined and extensive tests are currently under way. Because they are placed near critical structures inside the eye, there is concern that they may cause cataracts or glaucoma. If determined to be safe, intraocular implants may be used to treat people with too much nearsightedness or too much farsightedness for the LASIK technique.

RADIAL KERATOTOMY (RK)

Radial keratotomy was the first surgical procedure to be widely used to correct nearsightedness and, contrary to most people's understanding, does not involve the use of a laser. RK was invented in the Soviet Union in 1973 and was first performed in the United States in 1978. Over one million people around the world have been treated with RK.

Like excimer laser surgery, RK corrects nearsightedness by altering the shape of the cornea. The doctor makes a series of incisions in the periphery of the cornea. This increases the corneal curvature slightly where the incisions are made and decreases the curva-

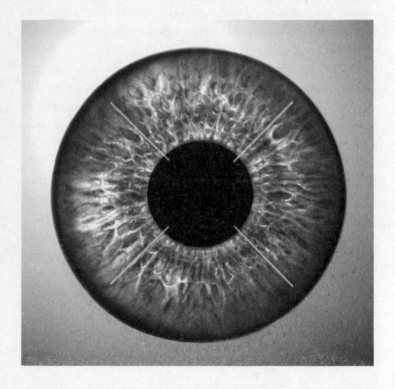

In radial keratotomy, a series of incisions is made in the cornea, causing the central cornea to flatten.

ture in the central portion of the cornea. The incisions are made in a radiating pattern, like the spokes on a bicycle wheel. By varying the number, length, depth, and location of these incisions, different amounts of nearsightedness can be corrected.

Although patient satisfaction with RK was very high, RK has now been largely replaced by excimer laser techniques and is seldom used today. LASIK and PRK produce results that are more accurate than RK and can treat a much wider range of focusing errors. Because of this greater accuracy, excimer laser patients are much less likely than RK patients to require a "touch-up" procedure. Also, RK patients experience side effects more commonly than do excimer laser patients. These side effects include starbursts when viewing a bright light against a dark background and fluctuation in vision throughout the day. RK patients, but not excimer laser patients, experience a temporary, reversible fluctuation in vision when at high altitudes. Pilots, mountain climbers, and skiers may be affected by this and should not have RK.

Astigmatic Keratotomy (AK)

Astigmatic keratotomy is a variation of RK, used to treat astigmatism. AK uses arc-shaped incisions in the cornea, whereas RK uses radial incisions, like the spokes of a wheel. Neither RK nor AK is performed with a laser.

AK is often performed in conjunction with RK and can also be performed in conjunction with excimer laser surgery. This is important, because not all excimer lasers can correct astigmatism, so excimer laser treatment of nearsightedness and farsightedness is occasionally combined with AK treatment of astigmatism. For mild or moderate astigmatism, AK's predictability is good but certainly not perfect. In most cases, it is more accurate to treat astigmatism with the excimer laser than to use AK.

Automated Lamellar Keratoplasty (ALK)

Performed from the 1970s until the mid-1990s, ALK was the forerunner to LASIK. In ALK, a keratome was used to peel back the front layers of the cornea, creating a flap, just as it is used in the LASIK procedure today. No tissue is permanently removed in the making of the flap; by making the flap, the doctor is able to work on the deeper tissue of the cornea. In ALK, the keratome was then used a second time to remove a small disc of cornea from under the flap, causing the central cornea to flatten and lessening nearsightedness. In LASIK, the tissue under the flap is instead removed using the excimer laser, which is much more precise.

ALK has been completely replaced by LASIK and is not performed anymore. In fact, ALK was never very popular because the second part of the procedure, removing the disc of tissue, was not adequately precise. However, without ALK we would probably not have LASIK today. LASIK is a combination of the flap technique of ALK with the precision of the excimer laser—a truly remarkable combination.

Because ALK has been performed since the 1970s, we have a long track record showing the safety of making corneal flaps. This is very important: because of

ALK, we know that there are no long-term safety problems from making corneal flaps!

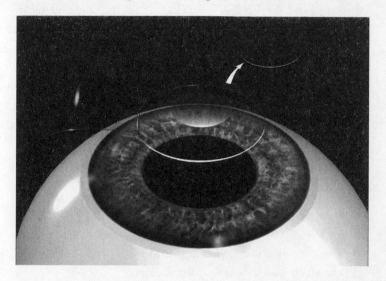

In automated lamellar keratoplasty for nearsightedness, the outer cornea is folded back and a small piece of tissue is removed.

ORTHOKERATOLOGY

Orthokeratology is not a surgical correction. Rather, it involves the use, over a course of months, of progressively flatter contact lenses to reduce the curvature of the cornea. After completing the course of treatment, the patient can see clearly for many hours without contact lenses or glasses. The patient continues to wear retainer contact lenses from two to seven times a week, usually while sleeping. Thus, successful orthokeratology results in the patient not needing contact lenses while awake, but wearing retainer contact lenses while asleep. If the patient stops wearing the retainer contact lens, his or her eye reverts to its original near-sightedness within one week.

Orthokeratology can temporarily correct mild near-sightedness, up to about that needing 3 diopter lenses, and works best in cases needing 2 diopters or less. It is not successful in all patients, because some patients develop a distortion of the cornea and have to discontinue treatment.

Orthokeratology is an option for patients with mild or very mild nearsightedness who may be able to tolerate contact lenses well but prefer not to wear them in public and do not want to undergo excimer laser treatment. People in certain occupations, such as policemen, firemen, or flight attendants, may use orthokeratology to pass their vision test requirements.

GLASSES AND CONTACT LENSES

Of course, most people have their nearsightedness, far-sightedness, and astigmatism corrected with glasses or contact lenses. Although it may be inconvenient to wear glasses or contact lenses, they do provide excellent vision in most cases. If you are satisfied using glasses or contact lenses, then there is no need for other forms of treatment. You should consider other treatments only if your glasses or contact lenses are uncomfortable or inconvenient or if you want good vision without glasses and contact lenses for personal or occupational reasons.

NO MORE READING GLASSES?

The most common focusing problem in the world is not nearsightedness, farsightedness, or astigmatism. Presbyopia (which means "old vision") is by far the most common focusing problem, because it affects every person beginning around age forty to fifty. Objects that are close to us require more focusing strength than objects that are far away. In young people, the crystalline lens changes shape (and thereby its focusing strength), depending on whether you are focusing on something in the distance or up close. This ability to change the focus from distance to near is known as accommodation. As we approach the age of forty to fifty, we begin to lose accommodation. The age-related loss of accommodation, which occurs in every person, is known as presbyopia.

Unfortunately, none of the techniques used to treat nearsightedness, farsightedness, or astigmatism also solves the problem of presbyopia.

People deal with presbyopia in several ways. The most common way of dealing with presbyopia is to use reading glasses, bifocals, or trifocals. Some people with presbyopia choose to have monovision, in which one eye is adjusted for distance and the other is adjusted for near. Monovision can be created with glasses, contact lenses, or with excimer laser treatment. Some people with mild nearsightedness, whose eyes are thereby naturally adjusted for near vision, simply remove their distance glasses to see clearly up close. However, these nearsighted people who also have presbyopia are unable to see clearly up close when their distance glasses or contact lenses are on.

Two techniques are now being tested that may provide relief for presbyopia:

Scleral expansion bands (SEB), manufactured by Presby, are four small pieces of plastic that are inserted into the white portion of the eye (the sclera). The procedure is performed as an outpatient, with the patient awake, and requires less than an hour. SEBs appear to improve the ability of people with presbyopia to read clearly up close, eliminating the need for reading glasses, without affecting the distance vision.

SEBs are currently being tested for safety and effectiveness by the FDA. If proven to be safe and effective over time, this technique could become extremely popular. People will be able to correct their distance vision with LASIK and could have SEBs to correct their age-limited near vision as well.

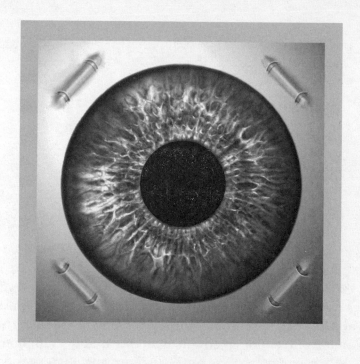

Four scleral expansion bands are placed in the white part of the eye, eliminating the need for reading glasses.

Another technique, known as anterior ciliary sclerostomy, is also being examined as a means of correcting presbyopia. Anterior ciliary sclerostomy involves making radiating incisions in the sclera. These incisions are similar to the incisions used in radial keratotomy (RK), except in RK the incisions are placed in the cornea. Anterior ciliary sclerostomy may not be satisfactory for most people because it appears to correct only a small amount of presbyopia.

THE FUTURE OF
LASER EYE SURGERY

What can we expect in the future for laser eye surgery? Certainly we can expect that laser techniques will undergo continual improvement. This should result from ongoing advances in laser and computer technology as well as an ever-improving understanding of how to optimally use these tools. As a result, in the future we should be able to help people who are not currently candidates for laser vision correction. Although excimer laser treatments presently produce excellent results, the future should yield even better results for more and more people.

Perhaps the most exciting advances lie in more advanced measurement and correction of complex imperfections in vision. Currently excimer lasers can correct nearsightedness, farsightedness, and astigmatism—just as do glasses and contact lenses. But what if we could use lasers to make people see better than is possible with glasses or contacts lenses?

Nearsightedness, farsightedness, and astigmatism are the major imperfections in the way light is focused. But all eyes, even those with 20/20 vision, have minor imperfections in the cornea, crystalline lens, and retina, causing minor distortions in the vision. These minor imperfections cannot be corrected with glasses or contact lenses but may be correctable in the future with lasers. Theoretically, by also correcting these imperfections, "perfect" vision could be improved from 20/20, possibly to 20/12.5, an improvement of over 35 percent! Our vision would not be as good as a hawk's, but it would be considerably better than human beings have ever experienced.

The problem lies in measuring these imperfections and then controlling the laser to precisely correct them. One approach uses corneal topography, which measures the tiny imperfections in the curvature of the front of the eye. A more ambitious approach uses wavefront analysis, which measures imperfections in light rays bounced off the back of the eye. Wavefront analysis has been successfully applied in astronomy to improve the resolution of telescopes. These measurement devices are linked directly to the computer that controls the laser. If these approaches are successful, laser vision correction may move beyond its current role—reducing the need for glasses and contact lenses—to a whole new realm. In the future, perhaps even those with 20/20 acuity will have laser correction to achieve a whole new level of vision.

||||||||||||||||||||||||||

AFTERWORD

MY OWN
EXPERIENCE AS A PATIENT

I began wearing glasses when I was twelve years old. Although I could see very well with them, I never liked the way I looked in glasses. Growing up in Florida, I loved to swim, but I couldn't see very well when I took my glasses off. Playing sports with glasses was often a problem, because my glasses would become foggy, sweaty, or would get knocked around.

I started wearing contact lenses during high school. These were much better than glasses for me. They didn't fog or get wet in the rain, and I had much better peripheral vision. Also, the contacts didn't cause the distortions that I always had with my glasses. My early contacts were hard lenses, and it did take a few miserable weeks to adjust to them. Occasionally a piece of dust would get under the lens and it felt like my eye was on fire.

During medical school at the age of twenty-two, I started to wear soft lenses, and these were better still.

The soft lenses were comfortable from the first day, and I could wear them almost all day long. However, after a long day of working in the hospital, my eyes would usually be very sore, and I would need to take the contacts out. Hopefully I had my glasses nearby. Some days my eyes would be so sore that I couldn't wear the contacts at all.

Wouldn't it be great, I often thought, if I didn't need these glasses or contacts? Growing up, I viewed my nearsightedness and astigmatism as my biggest handicap, so it wasn't surprising that after completing medical school, I specialized in ophthalmology and concentrated my practice on correcting vision focusing problems.

Day after day, year after year, my patients would tell me that correcting their nearsightedness and astigmatism was one of the best things that had ever happened to them. I treated my own brother and many of my closest friends, in each case with fantastic results. However, because of my relatively high amount of nearsightedness, I was never an excellent candidate for radial keratotomy, which was incredibly frustrating. I was, however, a good candidate for excimer laser correction, so when the procedure became available in the United States, I decided to have it myself.

I chose to have the LASIK technique because of the faster visual recovery. Also, because of my moderately high degree of nearsightedness, I thought that LASIK had a slightly better likelihood of providing a full correction.

I knew that there was no guarantee that I would obtain a perfect correction, but I also knew that there was a high probability that I would see well enough to do away with my glasses and contacts for most activities. Because I was over forty years old, I had been noticing some difficulty with near vision, though I hadn't yet started to use reading glasses or bifocals. I knew that excimer laser treatment would not solve this problem and that in the next several years I would begin to need reading glasses.

During the preoperative examination, my eyes were examined and my nearsightedness and astigmatism were measured. Corneal topography was performed. I was asked to read and sign a long document, which explained the technique, including what it could do and what could go wrong. The doctor also discussed the more common complications with me. Although I had gone over this with my own patients thousands of times, I still listened very carefully.

The procedure itself was very easy. First, my eye was washed out and numbing drops were put in. After lying down on the table, a speculum was placed in my eyelids to keep them open. All I could really see were several very bright lights. The doctor then created the thin flap with the keratome, which didn't hurt and took only a few seconds. I was then asked to look at a blinking light, and I heard the clicking noise of the laser. Again, there was no pain. During the course of the treatment, the blinking light became blurry and changed shape, but I was still able to look at it. The doctor then rinsed the eye and folded the flap back into place. The whole surgery had taken less than ten minutes.

A few minutes later, a stinging feeling began in the eye. I didn't take any pain medicine, because the stinging wasn't very bad, but someone else might have wanted to take a mild pain pill. After three or four hours, the stinging feeling went away. I put in the first of the eye drops, which I was told to continue using for a week.

The morning after my LASIK, I was stunned by how good my vision was. It wasn't perfect, but it was very, very good. It had improved so much in such a short time! I was able to drive myself the day after the procedure. Reading was a little strained during the first several weeks, and my vision would fluctuate somewhat during the day. During the first several weeks, I also experienced glare and halos around lights, but this gradually receded.

I returned to work three days after my procedure. After two weeks I felt very comfortable with my vision and resumed performing surgery.

During the next few months, my vision gradually became sharper. There was still some fluctuation; there were some times when the vision seemed sharper, and other times when it was less precise. During the first several months, my vision was particularly poor in dim light, and I experienced mild double vision with the left eye. These problems resolved after three to four months.

I am now able to work, drive, play sports, and go to movies without needing any glasses or contacts. My eyes are a lot less irritated now that I don't wear contacts; they are whiter and less sensitive to the sun. I can see well when I wake up in the morning, and swimming has become a lot more fun. I don't have to bother with all those contact lens solutions and don't have to worry about having an extra pair of glasses available. My clear vision is now part of me, instead of something I would put on and take off.

My young children, Jocelyn and Bryce, are very disappointed. They loved to give me a big kiss each morning and then pull off my glasses and throw them around, but there aren't any glasses anymore!

||||||||||||||||||||||||

APPENDIXES

Other Sources
of Information

American Academy of Ophthalmology
P.O. Box 7424
655 Beach Street
San Francisco, CA 94109

American Optometric Association
243 N. Lindbergh Boulevard
St. Louis, MO 63141

American Society of Cataract and Refractive Surgery
4000 Legato Road, Suite 850
Fairfax, VA 22033

International Society of Refractive Surgery
2215 Park Avenue
Minneapolis, MN 55404

Refractive Surgery Equipment Manufacturers

Aesculap-Meditec
Rustein 7
Heroldsberg, Germany 90562
011-49-911-518550

Alcon
6201 S. Freeway
Ft. Worth, TX 76434
817-293-0450

Autonomous Technologies
520 N. Semoran Boulevard, Suite 180
Orlando, FL 32807
407-282-1262

Bausch and Lomb
555 W. Arrow Highway
Claremont, CA 91711
800-496-7457

Intelligent Surgical Lasers (Escalon Medical)
4520 Executive Drive, Suite 1
San Diego, CA 92121
619-552-6700

KeraVision
48630 Milmont Drive
Fremont, CA 94538
510-353-3000

LaserSight
12249 Science Drive, Suite 160
Orlando, FL 32826
407-382-2700

Nidek
47651 Westinghouse Drive
Fremont, CA 94539
510-226-5700

Novatec Laser System
2237 Faraday Avenue
Carlsbad, CA 92008
619-438-6682

Presby Corporation
5910 North Central Expressway
Dallas, TX 75206
214-368-0200

Refractec
3 Jenner, Suite 140
Irvine, CA 92618
949-784-2600

Herbert Schwind GmbH
Main Part Str. 6
Kleinostheim, Germany 63801
011-49-6027-5080

Summit Technology
21 Hickory Drive
Waltham, MA 02154
617-890-1234

Sunrise Technologies
47257 Fremont Boulevard
Fremont, CA 94538
510-623-9001

Chiron-Technolas GmbH
Max-Planck Str. 6; Dornack Gem.
Aschheim, Germany 85609
011-49-89-9455140

VISX
3400 Central Expressway
Santa Clara, CA 95051
408-773-7000

GLOSSARY

It is hard to understand a technical subject such as excimer laser surgery without using specialized words. Here are definitions of some of the terms used in refractive surgery and in this book.

ablation: removal of tissue, for example, from the front surface of the cornea.

accommodation: the ability of the eye to change focus from distance to midrange to near; the loss of accommodation is known as presbyopia.

AK (see astigmatic keratotomy).

ALK (see automated lamellar keratoplasty).

amblyopia (lazy eye): a condition in which the eye structure is normal but the processing of visual information limits the visual acuity.

ametropia: a condition of imprecise focus, such as nearsightedness or farsightedness.

anterior ciliary sclerostomy: an experimental technique to treat presbyopia.

argon laser: a type of laser commonly used to treat glaucoma, retinal, and diabetic eye diseases.

astigmatic keratotomy (AK): a variation of radial keratotomy, in which incisions are made into the surface of the cornea to correct astigmatism.

astigmatism: asymmetrical focus of the light rays.

automated lamellar keratoplasty (ALK): a procedure for correcting nearsightedness or farsightedness in which a layer of cornea is cut, and sometimes an additional layer is removed.

axis: the direction of the astigmatism.

bilateral: pertaining to two sides; pertaining to both eyes.

cataracts: a clouding of the crystalline lens of the eye; if severe, surgical removal of the crystalline lens is needed.

central islands: a complication of excimer laser treatment in which the central corneal surface becomes raised.

CK (see conductive keratoplasty).

conductive keratoplasty: a technique to correct farsightedness that uses radio frequency energy; same as radio frequency keratoplasty.

contrast sensitivity: a measure of visual ability, specifically the ability to distinguish details under varying degrees of contrast.

cornea: the transparent tissue at the front of the eye.

corneal ring: a small plastic device placed in the cornea to correct nearsightedness; also known as the ICR, intrastomal corneal ring, or Intacs.

corneal topography: a computer-assisted technique for measuring the surface contours of the cornea.

crystalline lens: the hard tissue located just behind the iris, which focuses light rays.

decentration: a complication during excimer laser surgery in which the tissue is removed off center.

diopter: the measurement of a lens's ability to focus light rays. One diopter of focusing ability will focus parallel rays of light at one meter.

ectasia (see kerato-ectasia).

emmetropia: the normal condition of the eye in which the light rays focus on the retina.

epikeratophakia: a discontinued procedure for the correction of nearsightedness in which a lens is sewn onto the surface of the cornea.

epithelium: the thin, jellylike layer of cells on the surface of the cornea. In PRK, this tissue is removed and grows back in about three days.

excimer laser: an argon-fluorine gas laser that produces an ultraviolet beam used to remove corneal tissue accurately.

farsightedness (hyperopia): a focusing error in which the light rays are focused behind the retina. This results when the cornea and the crystalline lens together have too little focusing power for the length of the eye.

FDA (Food and Drug Administration): an agency of the federal government that monitors new medical devices and drugs.

flap and zap: the nickname for laser in-situ keratomileusis (LASIK), a procedure in which a flap is made in the cornea and excimer laser energy is then applied to tissue inside the cornea.

glaucoma: a disease characterized by abnormally high pressure within the eye.

haze: a complication of excimer laser surgery in which the cornea develops cloudiness.

hexagonal keratotomy: a discontinued procedure for the correction of farsightedness, involving making cuts into the cornea in the shape of a hexagon.

holmium laser: a laser used to correct farsightedness.

hyperopia (farsightedness): a focusing error in which the light rays are focused behind the retina. This results when the cornea and the crystalline lens together have too little focusing power for the length of the eye.

ICR (intrastromal corneal ring): a small plastic device placed in the cornea to correct nearsightedness; also known as corneal ring or Intacs.

informed consent: the legal process whereby a patient receives and acknowledges the risks, benefits, and alternatives to a medical procedure.

Intacs: the ICR (intrastromal corneal ring) manufactured by KeraVision.

intraocular implants: plastic lenses placed in front of or behind the iris to correct nearsightedness, farsightedness, or astigmatism.

intrastromal: within the cornea, as opposed to on the surface of the cornea.

intrastromal corneal ring (ICR): a small plastic ring used to correct nearsightedness. The ring is placed inside the edge of the cornea.

intrastromal lens: a clear lens placed within the cornea for correction of focusing abnormalities.

iris: the visible colored tissue inside the eye.

irregular astigmatism: irregular curvature of the cornea.

kerato-: of, or pertaining to, the cornea. From the Greek word for "cornea."

keratoconus: a disease of the cornea in which the central cornea becomes thinner and irregularly shaped.

kerato-ectasia: a bulging of the cornea, resulting from too much thinning.

keratome: the instrument used in creating the flap in the LASIK technique.

keratomileusis: an abandoned surgical procedure to correct nearsightedness in which a piece of the cornea is removed, reshaped, and reattached.

keratoplasty: surgical alteration of the cornea.

krypton laser: a type of laser used to treat retinal eye disease.

lamellar keratoplasty: a procedure for correcting nearsightedness or farsightedness in which a layer of cornea is cut, and sometimes an additional layer is cut and removed.

laser: a device that creates a beam of light that is perfectly synchronized and of the same wavelength.

laser in-situ keratomileusis (LASIK): a procedure in which a flap is made in the cornea and excimer laser energy is then applied to tissue inside the cornea; also known as "flap and zap."

laser thermal keratoplasty (LTK): an experimental procedure that uses a laser to heat portions of the cornea, resulting in the correction of farsightedness.

LASIK (see laser in-situ keratomileusis).

lazy eye (amblyopia): a condition in which the eye structure is normal but the processing of visual information limits the visual acuity.

lens: a device that focuses light rays.

LTK (see laser thermal keratoplasty).

micron: one millionth of a meter, or a thousandth of a millimeter; equivalent to about 39 millionths of an inch (also known as "micrometer").

monovision: adjusting the vision in one eye for distance and the other eye for near vision. This is an alternative to reading glasses and can be accomplished with contact lenses or with refractive surgery.

myopia (nearsightedness): a focusing error in which the light rays are focused in front of the retina. This results when the cornea and the crystalline lens together have too much focusing power for the length of the eye.

nearsightedness (myopia): a focusing error in which the light rays are focused in front of the retina. This results when the cornea and the crystalline lens together have too much focusing power for the length of the eye.

off-label: the use of an FDA-approved drug or medical device in a way that has not been explicitly approved by the FDA.

optic nerve: the nerve behind the eye that transmits visual information from the eye to the brain.

optical zone: in radial keratotomy, the area of the central cornea in which incisions are not placed.

orthokeratology: a technique for temporarily decreasing the curvature of the cornea using contact lenses.

overcorrection: a complication of excimer laser surgery in which too much tissue is removed from the cornea.

pachymeter: a device that measures the thickness of the cornea, usually by ultrasound.

PARK (see photoastigmatic refractive keratectomy).

PERK (prospective evaluation of radial keratotomy) study: a study funded by the National Institutes of Health that studied 435 patients who had radial keratotomy surgery beginning in 1982.

phakic: referring to the natural crystalline lens of the eye.

phakic intraocular implants: lenses placed into the eye in addition to the natural crystalline lens.

photoastigmatic refractive keratectomy (PARK): an excimer laser procedure to correct astigmatism, in which tissue is removed from the front surface of the cornea.

photorefractive keratectomy (PRK): an excimer laser surgical procedure to correct nearsightedness, in which tissue is removed from the surface of the cornea.

phototherapeutic keratectomy: an excimer laser surgical procedure in which tissue is removed from the surface of the cornea to remove scars and other irregularities.

presbyopia: the gradual loss of the ability to adjust the eye's focus that is a normal part of the aging process. This results in a loss of the ability to adjust focus from distant to nearby objects.

PRK (see photorefractive keratectomy).

progressive hyperopia: a complication of radial keratotomy in which a progressive flattening of the cornea occurs months or years after the procedure.

PTK (see phototherapeutic keratectomy).

pupil: the black opening in the iris that gets larger or smaller depending on the amount of light entering the eye.

radial keratotomy (RK): a surgical procedure for correcting nearsightedness, in which small incisions are made in the surface of the cornea.

radio frequency keratoplasty: a technique to correct farsightedness that uses radio frequency energy; same as conductive keratoplasty.

refraction: in ophthalmology, measuring the focus of the eye, usually by placing multiple test lenses in front of the eye.

refractive error: an inaccuracy in the focusing ability of the eye; includes nearsightedness, farsightedness, and astigmatism.

refractive surgery: the surgical correction of refractive errors.

regression: a complication of excimer laser surgery in which an initially favorable result changes in the direction of the original condition.

retina: the tissue in the back of the eye that receives the light rays.

RFK (see radio frequency keratoplasty).

RK (see radial keratotomy).

sclera: the white tissue that surrounds the eyeball.

scleral expansion band: a device, implanted into the white portion of the eye, that is being tested to correct presbyopia.

sclerostomy (see anterior ciliary sclerostomy).

SEB (see scleral expansion band).

thermal keratoplasty: a procedure to correct farsightedness and astigmatism in which heat is applied into the cornea; lasers are now being tested for this procedure, which is known as laser thermal keratoplasty.

topography: a computer-assisted technique for measuring the surface contours of the cornea.

transepithelial: a variation of photorefractive keratectomy in which the laser is used to remove the epithelium, the thin layer of cells on the surface of the cornea.

undercorrection: a complication of excimer laser surgery in which too little tissue is removed from the cornea.

visual acuity: the ability of the eye to resolve visual detail.

visual cortex: the area of the brain that processes the visual information from the eye.

vitreous humor: the gel-like substance that fills the space between the crystalline lens and the retina.

wavefront analysis: a technique for measuring complex imperfections in vision by using light bounced off the back of the eye.

wavelength: the distance between two identical, successive parts of a wave of light; responsible for the "color" of the light.

YAG (yttrium-aluminum-garnet) laser: a laser used in ophthalmology to cut transparent membranes.

ACKNOWLEDGMENTS

A tremendous amount of work has gone into producing this book, and it would not have been possible without help from many people. First and foremost, I would like to thank my wife, Jacqueline, who has lovingly understood the countless hours that I have worked on this book before and after my normal occupation of taking care of patients. I would like to thank my office staff—most of whom have trusted me to correct their own or their spouse's vision—for bringing zest and professionalism to everything they do. Diane Shader Smith and Mark Smith provided invaluable guidance during the early phases of the book, and Alison Schneider helped add depth and warmth to the manuscript. My publisher, Claire Ferraro, and editor, Cathy Repetti, had the vision to make this project possible. Most of all, I would like to thank my many patients who read the manuscript; your comments helped bring clarity and completeness to this book.

Index

ABOUT THE AUTHOR

ANDREW I. CASTER, M.D., has performed over twelve thousand procedures to correct nearsightedness, far-sightedness, and astigmatism. Dr. Caster is widely considered one of the most knowledgeable LASIK surgeons in the United States; he appears on many "Best LASIK Surgeon" and "Best Doctor" lists. Patients travel to Dr. Caster for the LASIK procedure from across the United States as well as from many other countries. A graduate of Harvard Medical School, Dr. Caster is a fellow of the American Academy of Ophthalmology and the American College of Surgeons. Dr. Caster is in practice in the Los Angeles, California, area with offices in Beverly Hills. You can visit with Dr. Caster at his Web site, www.castervision.com.